Getting the Board on Board

What Your Board Needs to Know About Quality and Patient Safety

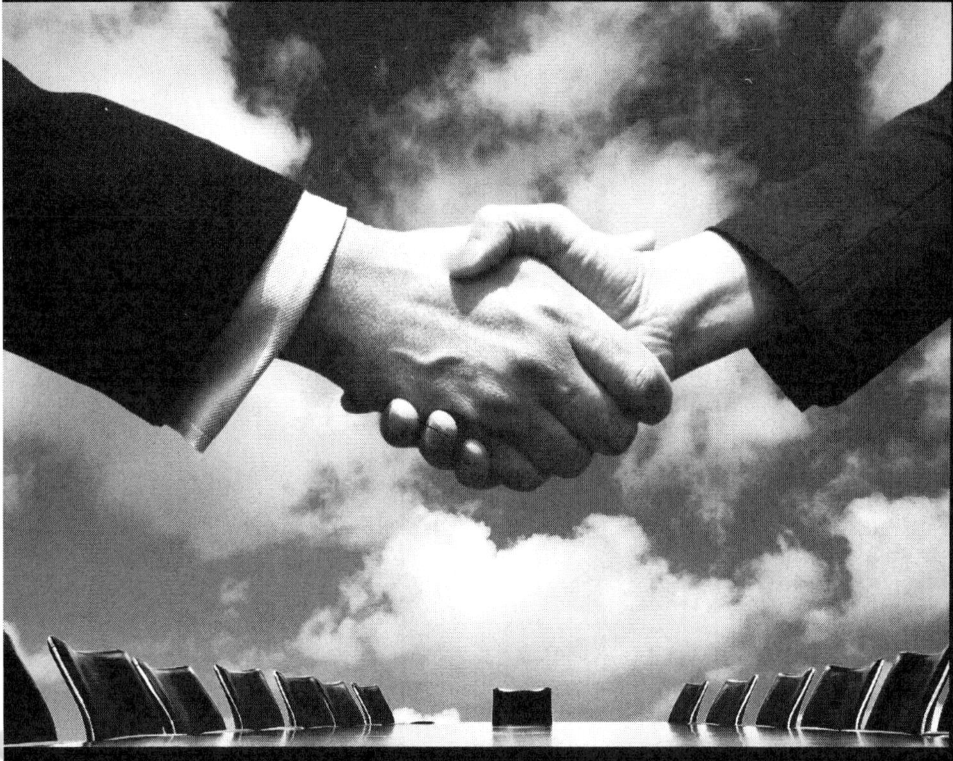

Second Edition

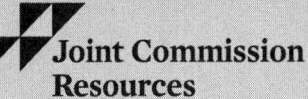
Joint Commission Resources

Senior Editor: Katie Byrne
Senior Project Manager: Cheryl Firestone
Manager, Publications: Lisa Abel
Associate Director, Production: Johanna Harris
Executive Director: Catherine Chopp Hinckley, Ph.D.
Joint Commission/JCR Reviewers: Patricia Adamski, Maureen P. Carr, Helen M. Fry, Catherine Chopp Hinckley, Jerod M. Loeb, Mark G. Pelletier, Paul M. Schyve, Gail Weinberger, Robert A. Wise, Frank S. Zibrat

Joint Commission Resources Mission
The mission of Joint Commission Resources (JCR) is to continuously improve the safety and quality of health care in the United States and in the international community through the provision of education, publications, consultation, and evaluation services.

Joint Commission Resources educational programs and publications support, but are separate from, the accreditation activities of The Joint Commission. Attendees at Joint Commission Resources educational programs and purchasers of Joint Commission Resources publications receive no special consideration or treatment in, or confidential information about, the accreditation process.

The inclusion of an organization name, product, or service in a Joint Commission Resources publication should not be construed as an endorsement of such organization, product, or service, nor is failure to include an organization name, product, or service to be construed as disapproval.

This publication is designed to provide accurate and authoritative information in regard to the subject matter covered. Every attempt has been made to ensure accuracy at the time of publication; however, please note that laws, regulations, and standards are subject to change. Please also note that some of the examples in this publication are specific to the laws and regulations of the locality of the facility. The information and examples in this publication are provided with the understanding that the publisher is not engaged in providing medical, legal, or other professional advice. If any such assistance is desired, the services of a competent professional person should be sought.

© 2011 The Joint Commission

Joint Commission Resources, Inc. (JCR), a not-for-profit affiliate of The Joint Commission, has been designated by The Joint Commission to publish publications and multimedia products. JCR reproduces and distributes these materials under license from The Joint Commission.

All rights reserved. No part of this publication may be reproduced in any form or by any means without written permission from the publisher.

Printed in the U.S.A. 5 4 3 2 1

Requests for permission to make copies of any part of this work should be mailed to
Permissions Editor
Department of Publications
Joint Commission Resources
One Renaissance Boulevard
Oakbrook Terrace, Illinois 60181
permissions@jcrinc.com

ISBN: 978-1-59940-550-6
Library of Congress Control Number: 2011920446

For more information about Joint Commission Resources, please visit http://www.jcrinc.com.

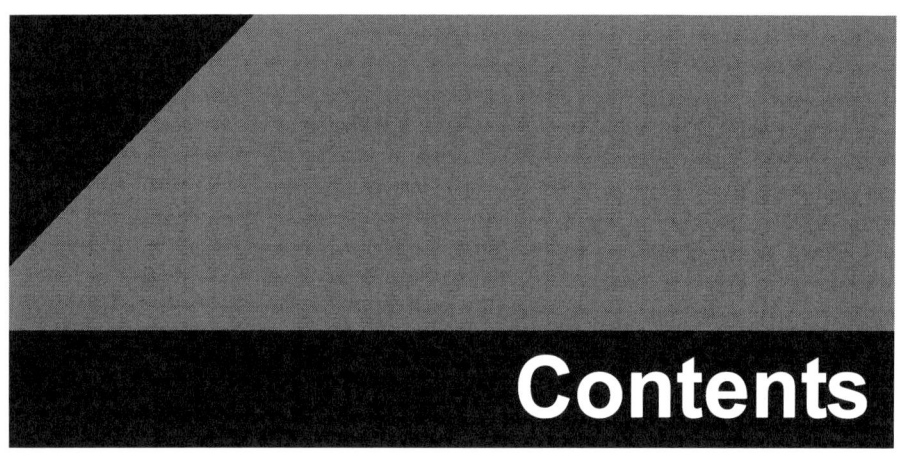

Contents

Introduction v

Chapter 1.
An Overview of Quality and Safety Issues Facing Health Care Organizations 1
Health Care Reform 1
Sentinel Events and Close Calls 15
Common Safety Areas of Concern 22
The Next Step 28

Chapter 2.
What You Need to Know About The Joint Commission 33
Accreditation, Certification, Standards, and Measures 34
Performance Measurement and the ORYX® Initiative 49
Patient Safety 53
Quality Check® 60
The Next Step 70

Chapter 3.
The Board's Role in Improving Quality and Safety 71
Promoting a Culture of Quality and Safety 73
Participating in Measurement and Improvement 85
Holding Management Accountable for Change 93
Addressing Quality and Safety in Board Meetings 95
The Next Step 97

Glossary 99

Index 103

Introduction

The U.S. health care industry is in a tumultuous and transformational state due to an unprecedented economic downturn, the need to improve the quality of health care, and government-mandated health care reform. Although the pool of insured Americans will increase by at least 32 million people over the next few years, reimbursement for health care services will decrease dramatically.[1] Experts estimate a decrease in reimbursement of about $200 billion over the next decade.[2] This decrease in reimbursement will force health care organizations to provide high-quality, competitive health care while maximizing productivity and reducing costs. Health care boards* are in a prime position to help navigate the changes as well as capitalize on the opportunities introduced by national health care reform legislation. At the same time, boards are also guiding their health care organizations through the worst recession since the Great Depression. Health care organizations that have survived the recession thus far have been able to cut costs while increasing productivity. But health care reform demands quality despite the fact that health care now has to be provided with fewer expenses and resources. Overall, to compete in the health care industry during this transformational phase, health care boards need to be prepared and informed while focusing on providing high-quality care that meets the expectations for reimbursement.

Today, board members retain as much responsibility for the quality and safety as for the financial surety of their organizations. In fact, a study from the Agency for Healthcare Research and Quality found that when governing boards are involved in

---

* The governing bodies of health care organizations may be known by a variety of names. In this book, the terms *board, board of trustees,* and *governing body* are used synonymously. The individuals serving on these boards are referred to as *board members* or *trustees.*

quality and safety, their hospitals' mortality rates decrease and performance in processes of care improves.³ Furthermore, insurers, purchasers, and patients* are using public reports of performance to make decisions about their provider preferences, and pay-for-performance programs are using these same reports to guide reimbursement and enforce the organizations' accountability to the public for their performance. Government and accrediting bodies require that trustees monitor quality within their organizations. Ultimate responsibility for the care and safety of patients rests with the governing body, and maintaining control of this aspect of governance takes time, commitment, and resources. "Deeply engaged leadership," starting with the board, is a crucial attribute of organizations demonstrating sustained progress in patient safety.⁴

Since The Joint Commission revised its Leadership standards and other influential organizations encouraged boards to have an increased role in patient safety and quality improvement, boards have responded positively. A recent survey of 722 chairpersons across U.S. health care organizations found the following results⁵:

- Sixty-three percent of hospital boards discuss quality improvement issues at each meeting, and this discussion comprises at least 20% of the agenda for more than half the boards.
- Three out of five hospital boards have a quality subcommittee.
- Seventy-two percent of hospital boards regularly review quality dashboards.
- More than half of hospital board members consider quality of care to be a top priority.

However, the same study indicates that only 32% of hospital boards have received any formal training in clinical quality.⁵ Even though financial incentives often provide leaders with the motivation to reach quality improvement goals, only 44% of boards include quality of care as one of the two most important criteria for evaluating the CEO's performance.⁵

This book will provide you, a hospital board member, with an overview of the issues you should be aware of (Chapter 1) and explain the Joint Commission's role

---

* Different settings refer in different ways to those they serve. In this book, the term *patient* includes residents, clients, and individuals served.

in helping organizations reduce risks and develop measures and processes to maximize quality and safety (Chapter 2). This book also provides real-world examples of how health care boards in hospitals across the country have taken the lead in making quality and safety top priorities in their organizations (Chapter 3). Whether you are just beginning your tenure or have participated on a governing board for some time, we hope that this book will assist you in carrying out your responsibilities as a board member and deepen your commitment to health care quality and patient safety.

These are two of the most important questions trustees can ask themselves: "If someone I loved were ill, would I want that person to receive care from the organization I govern? Would I myself want to receive care from that organization?"[6] If you are not sure what level of quality and safety your organization can provide, the answer to these questions is probably "no." There may be work to be done to change that—to a resounding "yes!"

Acknowledgments

We are grateful to the following people for their invaluable insights and perspectives:

- Kent Bottles, M.D., former vice president and chief medical officer, Iowa Health System, Des Moines
- Jeffrey Brickman, F.A.C.H.E., system senior vice president and president and chief executive officer, Provena Saint Joseph Medical Center, Joliet, Illinois
- Lee Carter, trustee, Cincinnati Children's Hospital Medical Center, Cincinnati
- Melissa Coleman, board member, Delnor-Community Hospital, Geneva, Illinois
- Maureen Connor, R.N., M.P.H., former vice president for quality improvement and risk management, Dana-Farber Cancer Institute, Boston
- Richard Davis, Ph.D., executive director of Johns Hopkins Medicine Center for Innovation in Quality of Patient Care, Baltimore
- Yosef D. Dlugacz, Ph.D., senior vice president, Krasnoff Quality Management Institute, and chief clinical quality, education, and research, North Shore–Long Island Jewish Health System, Great Neck, New York

- Wanda Gibbons, R.N., M.H.A., former vice president of patient care services and chief nursing officer, St. Vincent's Medical Center, Jacksonville, Florida
- John Hensing, M.D., executive vice president and chief medical officer, Banner Health, Phoenix
- John Hubbe, Pharm.D., J.D., vice president of medical and legal services, Delnor-Community Hospital, Geneva, Illinois
- William F. Jessee, M.D., F.A.C.M.P.E, F.A.C.P.M., former chair of the board of directors, Exempla Health System, Denver
- Vincent O'Reilly, vice chair, Dana-Farber Cancer Institute, Boston
- Lori Paine, R.N., M.S., director, patient safety, The Johns Hopkins Hospital, Baltimore
- Janet Porter, Ph.D., executive vice president and chief operating officer, Dana-Farber Cancer Institute, Boston
- William Varani, M.D., vice president of quality, Bon Secours Health System, Inc., Marriottsville, Maryland
- Saul N. Weingart, M.D., Ph.D., vice president for quality improvement and patient safety, Dana-Farber Cancer Institute, Boston
- Gary Yates, M.D., senior vice president and chief medical officer, Sentara Healthcare, Norfolk, Virginia

We also thank Meghan Pillow, R.N., for her diligence and patience in writing this book.

References

1. DeVore S.: Top 10 things hospitals need to know about health reform . . . but were afraid to ask. *Healthc Financ Manage* 64:44–45, Aug. 2010.
2. Kellis D.S.: Healthcare reform and the hospital industry: What can we expect? *J Healthc Manag* 55:283–296, Jul.–Aug. 2010.
3. Jiang H.J., Bass K., Fraser I.: Board oversight of quality: Any differences in process of care and mortality? *J Healthc Manag* 54:15–29, Jan.–Feb. 2009.
4. Institute for Healthcare Improvement: *Getting Started Kit: Governance Leadership How-to Guide* (Get Boards on Board). http://www.ihi.org/IHI/Programs/Campaign/BoardsonBoard.htm (accessed Feb. 7, 2011).
5. Jha A., Epstein A.: Hospital governance and the quality of care. *Health Aff (Millwood)* 29:182–187, Jan.–Feb. 2010.
6. The Governance Institute: *The Board's Role in Monitoring Quality.* La Jolla, CA: The Governance Institute, 2000.

Chapter 1

An Overview of Quality and Safety Issues Facing Health Care Organizations

Before you can become truly involved in promoting better quality and safety within your hospital, you and your fellow board members must understand the issues affecting the hospital and the health care field in general. Depending on their respective fields, one board member may be more familiar with legislation or financial concerns and another with medical advances. Familiarity with the quality and reform movement that has grown in recent years, an understanding of sentinel events and the need for performance measurement and improvement, and general knowledge regarding common vulnerabilities within hospitals can provide the foundation you need to put your hospital's needs and problems in context.

Health Care Reform

In 2010 Americans spent more than $2.6 trillion on health care services—that is, 17.6% of the gross domestic product.[1] To put this in perspective, Americans spent three times more on health care than on the defense budget and two times more on health care than on education.[1] Despite these seemingly exorbitant payments for health care, the United States ranked last out of six countries (the others being Australia, Canada, Germany, New Zealand, and the United Kingdom) in metrics of patient safety, patient access, efficiency, and equity.[1] In addition, the infant mortality rate, a common measure of a country's health and well-being, is much higher in the United States than in several countries that spend far less on health care. While the U.S. infant mortality rate is 6.14 per 1,000 live births, more than 45 other countries—including Monaco, Singapore, and Bermuda—have fewer infant deaths.[2] Furthermore, more than 59 million Americans do not have health insurance, dramatically decreasing their access to health care.[3] It is clear, then, that the health care industry faces several challenging goals: to decrease health care spending, to increase access to health care and health insurance, and to improve health care outcomes.

The goal of improving health care outcomes as well as the quality of care delivered by health care organizations has long been a subject of debate among health care organizations, clinicians, purchasers, politicians, insurers, and patients. Because increased attention has been given to the high number of common medical errors that occur during routine care and services, the U.S. government has become more involved in regulating the health care industry. Congress mandated sweeping changes to the industry in 2010 when it passed health care reform legislation (*see* Sidebar 1-1 below).

Sidebar 1-1. Affordable Health Care Act

This extensive legislation mandates the following[4-6]:

- All legal residents will be required to enroll in a qualified health plan by January 1, 2014, increasing the number of residents with health insurance coverage by 32 million.
- With more Americans required to obtain health insurance, costs associated with uncompensated care will be reduced by about $184.5 billion over 10 years.
- Medicare and Medicaid payments to hospitals are estimated to be cut by $149 billion (including reductions in diagnosis-related group payments, market basket updates, and disproportionate share hospital programs).
- The Department of Health & Human Services secretary will explore alternative methods, such as health courts and early offer programs, to resolve medical liability claims ($50 million to be spent over five years).
- Health care organizations with the highest readmission rates can participate in a five-year Medicare pilot program starting in 2011 to apply evidence-based interventions to reduce readmissions (priority is given to small community hospitals, rural hospitals, and organizations caring for medically underserved populations).
- Companies with 50 or more full-time employees that don't provide affordable health insurance will be penalized; the employees will receive affordability credits for health insurance.

(continued on page 3)

Sidebar 1-1. Affordable Health Care Act (continued)

- The Centers for Medicare & Medicaid Services (CMS) and the Agency for Healthcare Research and Quality will be given $75 million over five years to develop quality measures.
- A physician comparison database (similar to *Hospital Compare* [see more about *Hospital Compare* on page 7], but for physicians) will be made available to the public, requiring increased physician quality reporting.
- The CMS payment system will shift to pay for value-based services rather than for the number of services provided (in an effort to reduce unnecessary tests, procedures, and other services).
- Hospitals with higher-than-expected, risk-adjusted 30-day readmission rates for certain conditions (such as heart attack, heart failure, and pneumonia) will receive reduced payments.
- Hospitals with higher-than-expected, risk-adjusted rates for hospital-acquired conditions will face financial penalties. (In 2015 CMS will add a 1% penalty to hospitals in the top quartile of national risk-adjusted rates for hospital-acquired conditions for an applicable period in a fiscal year.)
- The Center for Medicare and Medicaid Innovation will be created within CMS to test and implement innovative reimbursement and service delivery models. Pilot programs are anticipated to test the effectiveness of bundled payments and accountable care organizations in reducing costs, improving quality, and providing financial rewards to health care systems:
  - Bundled payments will cover services provided from 3 days before admission to 30 days after discharge for inpatient and outpatient care, physician services, post-acute care, and any other services deemed appropriate by the Health & Human Services secretary.
  - Accountable care organizations provide low-cost and high-quality care by coordinating physician and hospital services.
- To maintain tax-exempt status, hospitals must conduct a community health needs assessment once every three years. In addition, hospitals must report to the Internal Revenue Service annually on how they are meeting identified community needs, create a financial assistance policy, and put forth "reasonable" effort to determine whether a patient qualifies for charity care.
- Hospitals need to make the prices for all items and services provided available to the public, including each Medicare Severity-Diagnosis Related Group.

As the requirements of health reform legislation unfold over the next few years, it is imperative that board members stay one step ahead so that they can help their organizations plan for the increased number of insured patients, decreased payments from Medicare and Medicaid, and opportunities for quality improvement programs afforded by the legislation.

The Joint Commission

The Joint Commission's mission is to continuously improve health care for the public, in collaboration with other stakeholders, by evaluating health care organizations and inspiring them to excel in providing safe and effective care of the highest quality and value. To accomplish this mission, The Joint Commission provides the following programs and services:

- Accreditation, which includes the establishment of standards as well as patient-centered on-site evaluations
- Performance measurement, through the development and implementation of standardized core measures for hospitals (the ORYX® initiative), accountability measures, and the performance-improving Strategic Surveillance System (S3)
- Patient safety efforts, including the development and implementation of National Patient Safety Goals, the maintenance of the Sentinel Event Database, and the establishment of the Center for Transforming Healthcare*
- Information dissemination to both the public and the health care field via its Quality Check® Web site at http://www.qualitycheck.org, which contains performance data, accreditation status, standards compliance history, compliance with the National Patient Safety Goals and performance measures, and distinctive achievements for accredited hospitals
- Public policy initiatives addressing topics such as nurse staffing, emergency preparedness, emergency department overcrowding, pay-for-performance, organ donation, medical liability reform, and health care professional education

In 2009 The Joint Commission established the Center for Transforming Healthcare to address the health care industry's most critical and complicated safety problems

---

* Publication and dissemination of the *Sentinel Event Alert* newsletter are described in detail in Chapter 2.

using Robust Process Improvement™ (RPI).[7] RPI incorporates Lean Six Sigma, change management, and other tools and methods for highly reliable outcomes.[7] The blended approach offered by Lean Six Sigma incorporates the following tools:

- Lean Thinking: Focuses on customer satisfaction by way of increasing value and reducing wasted time, resources, and money[7]
- Six Sigma: A statistical model that measures a process for potential defects[7]
- Change management: Principles designed to increase the success and accelerate the implementation of organizational change efforts

The Center has used these RPI methods to develop highly reliable quality solutions for hand-off communications, hand hygiene compliance, surgical site infections, and wrong-site surgery; more topics will be covered in future projects. To further simplify the process of solving safety issues, the Center created the Targeted Solutions Tool™, an online application that walks organizations through a step-by-step process for measuring performance, identifying barriers to excellent performance, and implementing tested solutions.[7] Each hospital will access the Targeted Solutions Tool for these and future projects through its secure *Joint Commission Connect*™ extranet site. All organization data, identified root causes, and suggested solutions for resolving safety issues will remain completely confidential.

National Quality Forum

One of the federal government's most highly visible forays into the quality of care arena was the 1997 formation of the President's Advisory Commission on Consumer Protection and Quality in the Health Care Industry. Composed of 32 members representing consumers, health care workers and professionals, provider organizations, state and local governments, and various health care experts, the commission was charged with advising the president about changes in the field and recommending ways to improve and ensure the value and quality of health care as well as to protect patients and health care workers. The consensus report published by the commission in 1998 suggested steps for creating a "national commitment to improving health care quality."[8] One of these steps was the formation of a quality forum.

The National Quality Forum (NQF), a not-for-profit membership organization, was created in 1999 to develop and implement a national strategy for health care quality measurement and reporting. Its members, drawn from many areas of health care, include providers, insurers, employers, consumer groups, professional associations, accrediting bodies (including The Joint Commission), researchers, and labor unions. NQF endorses national quality measures and promotes the use of evidence-based quality information to develop preferred practices for all types of health care settings. In February 2006, NQF merged with the National Committee for Quality Health Care, an organization of health industry leaders focusing on quality improvement. NQF currently focuses on bringing together diverse efforts to improve health care quality according to the following national priorities[9]:

- Patient and family engagement
- Safety
- Care coordination
- Palliative and end-of-life care
- Equitable access
- Elimination of overuse
- Population health
- Infrastructure supports

In addition, NQF maintains its focus on safety by creating and updating a list of serious reportable events in health care. Currently, 28 adverse events are considered to be serious, largely preventable, and of concern to both the public and health care providers. Many states use NQF's 28 serious reportable events as the basis for the list of adverse events that should be reported. Furthermore, NQF endorsed a set of 34 safe practices (or voluntary consensus standards) that clinical care settings can use to reduce the risk of harm to patients. To view the NQF–endorsed measures or to learn more about NQF's national priorities, go to http://www.qualityforum.org.

Centers for Medicare & Medicaid Services

Given that the Medicare program reimburses health care providers for more than $460 billion in services every year, CMS has a significant role when it comes to mandating that patients receive high-quality health care.[10] CMS also serves as a national public reporting system for adverse events because hospitals are required to report whether patients contracted a hospital-acquired condition during their stay.[11] In 2008 CMS chose 10 hospital-acquired conditions that would no longer be reimbursed at the higher Medicare rates, essentially stating that it would no longer pay for substandard care. The 10 categories of so-called "never events" are shown in Table 1-1, page 8.[11]

CMS also created the *Hospital Compare* Web site, which posts data regarding hospitals' performance on certain process-of-care and outcomes-of-care measures relative to that of other hospitals in their respective states and in the nation. Hospitals are eligible for a payment incentive if they report their performance data to CMS for *Hospital Compare*. The process-of-care measures focus on a hospital's effectiveness in treating heart attack, heart failure, pneumonia, and children's asthma and in preventing infections after surgery. (For 2011, CMS also will collect and report data on how well hospitals are treating strokes.) The outcomes-of-care measures include readmission rates and mortality rates for patients who have suffered a heart attack, heart failure, or pneumonia. Furthermore, CMS reports measures on a hospital's use of medical imaging tests (mammograms, magnetic resonance imaging, and computed tomography scans) for outpatients, with the goals of reducing patients' exposure to radiation and following up appropriately with test results. Finally, *Hospital Compare* reports the results of a national survey, *Hospital Consumer Assessment of Healthcare Providers and Systems*, which asks patients about their recent hospital visit. Survey questions may target patients' opinions about how well the nurses and physicians communicated, how effectively their pain was controlled, and whether they would recommend the hospital to someone else.

Health care reform legislation has engendered plans to add quality data regarding hospital-acquired conditions to the *Hospital Compare* Web site.[6] For more information about *Hospital Compare* or to look up various hospitals' performance ratings, visit http://www.hospitalcompare.hhs.gov.

Institute of Medicine Reports

Two classic reports issued by the Institute of Medicine's Committee on the Quality of Health Care in America focused attention on patient safety, a key component of high-quality care for the past two decades. The first report, *To Err Is Human: Building a Safer Health System*, which was published in 1999, estimated that as many as 98,000 people die in hospitals every year as a result of preventable medical errors. Adverse drug events, wrong-site surgery, suicides, restraint-related injuries and deaths, falls, burns, pressure ulcers, and mistaken patient identities were among

Table 1-1. Nonreimbursable Hospital-Acquired Conditions

1. Foreign object retained after surgery
2. Air embolism
3. Blood incompatibility
4. Category III and IV pressure ulcers
5. Falls and trauma
   - Fractures
   - Dislocations
   - Intracranial injuries
   - Crushing injuries
   - Burns
   - Electric shock
6. Manifestations of poor glycemic control
   - Diabetic ketoacidosis
   - Nonketotic hyperosmolar coma
   - Hypoglycemic coma
   - Secondary diabetes with ketoacidosis
   - Secondary diabetes with hyperosmolarity
7. Catheter-associated urinary tract infection
8. Vascular catheter–associated infection
9. Surgical site infection following these procedures:
   - Coronary artery bypass graft mediastinitis
   - Bariatric surgery
     — Laparoscopic gastric bypass
     — Gastroenterostomy
     — Laparoscopic gastric restrictive surgery
   - Orthopedic surgery
     — Spine
     — Neck
     — Shoulder
     — Elbow
     — Total knee replacement
     — Hip replacement
10. Deep vein thrombosis/pulmonary embolism

Source: Centers for Medicare & Medicaid Services, 2010.

the most common errors listed. The report outlined a comprehensive strategy by which government, health care providers, industry, and consumers could reduce preventable medical adverse events and set a minimum goal of 50% reduction in errors during the following five years.[12]

The second report, *Crossing the Quality Chasm: A New Health System for the 21st Century*, which was released in 2001, addressed restructuring the health care system as a whole (including delivery and payment mechanisms) to provide better patient care and to make the best use of available resources.[13] The report made recommendations for bridging the "chasm" between the existing health care environment and a more ideal one. The proposed focus was on chronic conditions, which demand more resources than acute episodic care, and the goal for all proposed changes was to have care that meets the following six "Aims for Improvement"[13]:

1. Safety
2. Effectiveness
3. Patient-centeredness
4. Timeliness
5. Efficiency
6. Equity

Going a step further, Donald Berwick, M.D., founder of the Institute for Healthcare Improvement (IHI), concluded in his "user's manual" for the report that the quality of professional work, delivery systems, hospitals, and policies should be judged according to individual patient experience.[14]

The *Quality Chasm* report highlighted six challenges for health care organizations[13]:

1. Redesigning care processes to better serve chronically ill patients across settings, between clinicians, and over time
2. Using information technology to automate clinical information and make it accessible to patients and clinicians
3. Managing the ever-increasing advances in methods/techniques and ensuring that health care professionals are competent to use them
4. Coordinating care across conditions, settings, and services over time
5. Working to build more effective multidisciplinary teams

6. Incorporating process and outcome measures into day-to-day activities

Both publications became foundations for the ensuing push to improve patient safety in all health care settings. The two reports also emphasized that the majority of errors result from faulty systems and processes rather than from the actions of specific individuals. They concluded that the only way to reduce errors is to change the systems and processes themselves.

The Leapfrog Group

One of the recommendations of *To Err Is Human* was that large companies use employer purchasing power to promote advances in health care quality and safety. This provided a basis for the founding of The Leapfrog Group in late 2000. Composed of a still-growing list of Fortune 500 companies and other large private and public health care purchasers, the group aims to initiate improvements in the safety, quality, and affordability of health care by recognizing and rewarding providers who make significant strides in these areas. The Leapfrog Hospital Rewards Program measures performance in five areas of effectiveness and affordability:

1. Coronary artery bypass graft
2. Percutaneous coronary intervention
3. Acute myocardial infarction
4. Community-acquired pneumonia
5. Deliveries/neonatal care

Data are collected through the group's Hospital Quality and Safety Survey or through the Joint Commission's ORYX vendors; hospitals that demonstrate excellence and/or exhibit improvement in these areas are rewarded.

The Leapfrog Group's Hospital Quality and Safety Survey asks hospitals to voluntarily submit data on four quality/safety practices[15]:

1. Computerized provider order entry
2. Evidence-based hospital referral (experience with high-risk treatments)
3. Intensive care unit staffing by physicians experienced in critical care medicine
4. Leapfrog Safe Practices Score (based on NQF–endorsed safe practices)

The results from this survey are available to member employers and consumers to help them make informed choices regarding health care providers.

The Leapfrog Group participates in many initiatives with other organizations as well. For example, it provides technical support to the national Rewarding Results initiative, which is aimed at helping payers, health plans, employers, and others develop ways (both monetary and nonmonetary) to reward physicians and hospitals for high-quality care. Rewarding Results is sponsored by the Robert Wood Johnson Foundation and the California HealthCare Foundation.

Institute for Healthcare Improvement

Many and varied quality and safety initiatives have been introduced by government agencies, accrediting bodies, professional associations, and individual health care systems. In December 2004 IHI launched the 100,000 Lives Campaign, through which it worked with other organizations to disseminate improvement tools and support expertise throughout the United States. The goal of this national patient safety initiative was to help save 100,000 lives before June 2006 by accelerating the pace of improvement in hospital care through the consistent implementation of proven lifesaving interventions. Many groups—including Agency for Healthcare Research and Quality, American College of Physicians, American Medical Association, CMS, The Joint Commission, National Association for Healthcare Quality, National Patient Safety Foundation, and Veterans Health Administration—endorsed the campaign. Table 1-2, page 12, lists the campaign interventions.

From December 2006 to December 2008, IHI led the 5 Million Lives Campaign to maintain the gains that were established in the 100,000 Lives Campaign, to enroll additional hospitals, and to promote the adoption of six new interventions. One of these new interventions is to get boards "on board" by defining and disseminating new and leveraged processes for hospital boards of directors to dramatically improve their effectiveness in accelerating the improvement of care.[16] The other new interventions are also listed in Table 1-2.

IHI provides several resources, including a how-to guide, to help governance leadership get involved in quality improvement and patient safety at http://www.ihi.org/IHI/Programs/Campaign/BoardsonBoard.htm (*see* Table 1-3, page 13).

> **Table 1-2. IHI 100,000/5 Million Lives Campaign Interventions**
>
> **Interventions from the 100,000 Lives Campaign**
> - Delivering reliable, evidence-based care for acute myocardial infarction to prevent deaths
> - Preventing adverse drug events by implementing medication reconciliation practices—a formal process of identifying the most accurate list of all medications a patient is taking; comparing it with physicians' admission, transfer, and/or discharge orders; notifying the physician of discrepancies; documenting needed changes; and providing a list of medications to the patient on discharge
> - Preventing central line infections by implementing a series of interdependent, scientifically grounded processes
> - Preventing surgical site infections by reducing risk factors and optimizing evidence-based processes of care
> - Preventing ventilator-associated pneumonia by implementing a series of interdependent, scientifically grounded processes
>
> **Interventions Added During the 5 Million Lives Campaign**
> - Preventing methicillin-resistant *Staphylococcus aureus* (MRSA) infection by reliably implementing scientifically proven infection control practices throughout the hospital
> - Reducing harm from high-alert medications, starting with a focus on anticoagulants, sedatives, narcotics, and insulin
> - Involving health care boards in the effort to define and spread new and leveraged processes to accelerate quality improvement
> - Reducing surgical complications by reliably implementing the changes in care recommended by the Surgical Care Improvement Project
> - Preventing pressure ulcers by reliably using science-based guidelines for prevention of this serious and common complication
> - Delivering reliable, evidence-based care for congestive heart failure to reduce readmissions

A Growing Focus on Board Responsibility

Consumers, government agencies, purchasers, insurers, and accrediting bodies are increasing their demands for health care organizations to be held accountable for the care they provide. Transparency, in the form of publicly available performance

> **Table 1-3. Board Checklist for Quality Improvement and Patient Safety**
>
> The Institute for Healthcare Improvement (IHI) recommends six actions for all boards to engage them in quality improvement and patient safety.[16]
>
> 1. Set aims (for example, to reduce unnecessary mortality and harm).
> 2. Get data and hear stories (for example, review quality dashboards at each board meeting and provide patient-specific stories to board members to put a "human face" on harm data).
> 3. Establish and monitor system-level measures (identify a small number of organizationwide measures of patient safety, such as facilitywide harm and risk-adjusted mortality).
> 4. Change the environment, policies, and culture to encourage respect, fairness, and justice.
> 5. Learn about and develop capability as a board to improve quality and patient safety.
> 6. Establish executive accountability for clear quality improvement targets.
>
> **Source:** Adapted from the Institute for Healthcare Improvement, *Protecting 5 Million Lives from Harm*, http://www.ihi.org/IHI/Programs/Campaign/Campaign.htm?TabId=0 (accessed Jan. 5, 2011).

data, has become increasingly mandatory so that patients and purchasers can compare providers and choose those that deliver the most value. As of November 2009, 27 states and the District of Columbia have passed legislation that requires health care organizations to report adverse events to state agencies.[17] Many states use NQF's 28 serious reportable events as the basis for the list of adverse events that should be reported. In addition, public reporting of health care–associated infection data is now mandatory in at least 25 states, and many others have similar legislation pending.[18] However, the lack of standardization in terminology and reporting methods limits the usefulness of the collected data for comparisons and identification of trends. Health care systems have an opportunity to become accountable for the care they provide, to help patients learn more about their conditions as a supplement to understanding the performance measures, and to use public reporting to foster process-of-care and outcome-improvement initiatives.[19]

The demand for accountability does not end with administrative leaders of hospitals; governing boards have also been brought into the mix. The Public Company Accounting Reform and Investor Protection Act of 2002, also known as the Sarbanes-Oxley Act, was passed in response to corporate scandals at some prominent companies. This act set forth new requirements for the governance of for-profit companies, but ripples have been felt throughout the nonprofit sector as well.

The following provisions of the act apply to nonprofit organizations[20]:

- Board members should be "independent," meaning free from any relationship with the hospital that could cause conflicts of interest. Trustees who are appointed to governance-related committees such as the audit committee or compensation committee *must* be independent.
- Requirements for executive compensation and "perks" include the return of bonuses or other compensation paid based on good financial performance when there is misconduct or a failure to comply with financial reporting standards. Loans or other "extensions of credit" to directors and senior officers are expressly forbidden.

Information on important events and transactions such as cancellation of significant contracts or incurrence of significant debt and defaults must be made available to investors/consumers. The CEO and chief financial officer (CFO) must certify the accuracy of financial statements and other information filed by the company with the Securities and Exchange Commission. The CFO and other senior financial officers must adopt a code of ethics.

Health care organizations across the country have used the Sarbanes-Oxley Act as a road map to evaluate and overhaul their own governance practices. Many hospitals have aligned themselves with the requirements concerning conflicts of interest, external and internal audits, and board independence.[20-22] They see this effort as a proactive approach to avoiding future financial problems and to anticipating similar laws that will be aimed at nonprofit organizations. In fact, at least 17 states are considering legislation to extend the Sarbanes-Oxley Act's provisions to nonprofits.[23]

Patient Involvement in Care

One of the recommendations of the Institute of Medicine's report *To Err Is Human: Building a Safer Health System* was that patients should be viewed as members of the health care team and as actively involved in the process of care.[8] Since then, federal agencies, national organizations concerned with health care quality, statewide safety coalitions, professional specialty associations, consumer groups, and health care providers have produced brochures and other materials advising patients what they can do to avoid errors and harm.[24] For example, the Agency for Healthcare Research and Quality's *20 Tips to Help Prevent Medical Errors* and the Joint Commission's *Speak Up: Help Prevent Errors in Your Care* program are intended to inform the public about how patients can help ensure their own safety.[25,26]

The Joint Commission's *YOU: The Smart Patient: An Insider's Handbook for Getting the Best Treatment*, coauthored with Michael F. Roizen, M.D., and Mehmet C. Oz, M.D., was published in early 2006; two weeks later, it was featured in the *New York Times* best sellers list. The book has sold more than 250,000 copies, received a nomination for a Quill Award, and been profiled on the television programs *Oprah* and *Good Morning America*. It has been featured in dozens of magazines and newspapers, including *Glamour, USA Today, Reader's Digest, Good Housekeeping,* and *Esquire.*

As discussed in *YOU: The Smart Patient*, patients are increasingly taking responsibility for managing their care as they use the Internet and other resources to identify appropriate treatments, health care settings, and physicians.[27]

This overview of the current quality/safety landscape is by no means comprehensive. Regulations and requirements, issues of concern, and improvement initiatives are constantly evolving, and board members need to make a concerted effort to familiarize themselves with what is happening in the field and how it affects their hospitals. Of course, they also need to know what is happening within their hospitals in terms of patient safety and overall improvement efforts.

Sentinel Events and Close Calls

A high-risk area in a health care organization may often go unnoticed until something actually goes wrong. A *sentinel event*—defined as an unexpected occurrence involving death or serious physical or psychological injury, or risk thereof—triggers an immediate investigation. The board should require that it be informed about sentinel event investigations and their outcomes. (Sentinel events are covered in more detail in Chapter 2 beginning on page 54.)

Sentinel events are not the same as medical errors: sentinel events are not always caused by medical errors, and medical errors do not always result in sentinel events. The following are the top 10 types of sentinel events reported* to The Joint Commission, in decreasing order of frequency[28]:

1. Wrong-site surgery
2. Delay in treatment
3. Operative and postoperative complications
4. Unintended retention of foreign body
5. Patient suicide
6. Patient fall
7. Other unanticipated event
8. Medication errors
9. Criminal event
10. Perinatal death/loss of function

Sometimes errors that might threaten the life or function of a patient are caught and corrected before they actually cause harm. This type of situation is considered a *close call*, defined as any process variation that did not affect the patient's outcome but for which a recurrence carries a significant chance of a serious adverse outcome. The investigation of these types of events can yield valuable information.

Reporting and Investigating Adverse Events

To make care and services as safe as possible, hospitals depend on staff reports of errors that do occur—whether they cause sentinel events or are close calls—so that systems can be reviewed and revised as necessary. As noted in the Institute of Medicine reports discussed earlier, most errors are caused by faulty systems that either allow mistakes or don't protect against them. Latent system failures caused by faulty design, maintenance, operation, or hospital error exist long before any error occurs. For example, many drug names have similar spellings and pronunciations but are used to treat completely different conditions. Therefore, a process for receiving verbal orders that does not include a step in which the nurse or pharma-

---

* The reporting of most sentinel events to The Joint Commission is voluntary and represents only a small proportion of actual events. Therefore, these data are not an epidemiologic data set, and no conclusions should be drawn about the actual relative frequency of events or trends in events over time.

cist taking the order reads back the complete medication order for verification may set the stage for an adverse drug event.

Hospitals may also choose to report errors and/or sentinel events to outside entities that can provide additional resources for addressing system problems. For example, The Joint Commission's Sentinel Event Policy (covered in more detail in Chapter 2) specifies certain types of events that are reviewable by The Joint Commission when experienced by a health care organization. The policy encourages hospitals to report sentinel events voluntarily. Adverse events and identified root causes are then entered into the Sentinel Event Database, which provides statistics that show causes, trends, settings, and outcomes.

When an error or adverse event is reported, the hospital needs to determine what went wrong through a root cause analysis. This process helps the staff examine a system's components, how the components relate to each other, and at what point the system broke down. A team that performs a root cause analysis first determines exactly what occurred and then asks why it occurred (that is, what were the immediate events or factors that contributed to the error?). Next, team members look for the underlying causes of those immediate events or factors, probing through as many layers of the system as necessary to find the most basic cause(s). Only after these root causes have been identified can effective action be taken to revise processes, ensuring that similar errors do not recur.

Taking a Proactive Approach

The examination and repair of faulty systems should not be limited to reactive situations after an adverse event. Many steps—such as improving access to information, standardizing and simplifying processes, and providing appropriate training for staff—can be taken proactively to help prevent errors. Two of the most far-reaching strategies are to create a culture that focuses on safety and quality and to improve communication throughout the hospital.

Building a Culture of Safety and Quality. Most high-risk industries (for example, the aviation industry) have reduced adverse events by creating cultures in which safe behaviors are rewarded and disciplinary systems allow employees to report their mistakes. Accurate error reporting by frontline staff is crucial to identifying system problems that need to be addressed. However, the corporate cultures of many health care organizations do not encourage this type of reporting. Traditional, hierarchical cultures tend to have punitive environments in which staff members are afraid to admit their own errors or report someone else's—particularly if the other person holds a higher-ranking position. A culture of safety and quality is patient centered and focuses on a proactive, multidisciplinary approach to continuously improving processes and preventing errors and adverse outcomes.

⊠ Standards in Practice ⊠

Creating a hospitalwide patient safety program is required by Leadership (LD) **Standard LD.04.04.05**, Element of Performance (EP) 1.

Standard LD.04.04.05 The hospital has an organizationwide, integrated patient safety program within its performance improvement activities.*

* **Source:** *2011 Comprehensive Accreditation Manual for Hospitals*. Please see the most current version of your organization's comprehensive accreditation manual for the most current standards and EPs.

Leaders, including board members, need to be the greatest proponents for this type of culture, working to build collaborative, nonconfrontational relationships between managers and all levels of staff.[29] They must emphasize that all information—positive or negative—is welcome and necessary so the hospital can learn the best ways to provide care. Staff members need to know that they will not be blamed either for their own mistakes or for close calls, or for pointing out the mistakes or close calls of others. Close calls afford opportunities to identify and correct problems before any adverse event.

⊠ Standards in Practice ⊠

A safety culture is referred to in **Standard LD.03.01.01**: Leaders create and maintain a culture of safety and quality throughout the hospital.*

* **Source:** *2011 Comprehensive Accreditation Manual for Hospitals*. Please see the most current version of your organization's comprehensive accreditation manual for the most current standards and EPs.

Improving Communication. Cultural, language, and communication barriers can lead to misunderstandings between health care providers and patients and their families, which in turn can result in adverse events and process problems such as misunderstood orders, wrong or missed doses of medication, and disruption of care continuity from one setting to another. Health literacy problems, which often go unrecognized and unaddressed by health care practitioners, undermine the ability of health care organizations to comply with the intent of the accreditation standards and safety goals designed to protect patients. In 2011 The Joint Commission updated several standards to emphasize the importance of maintaining effective communication between patients and health care providers (the box below lists these revised standards).

⊠ Standards in Practice ⊠

For 2011 The Joint Commission has updated the following standards to emphasize the importance of effective communication between patients and health care providers. Several other current standards support effective communication, cultural competence, and patient- and family-centered care.*

Standard PC.02.01.21 The hospital effectively communicates with patients when providing care, treatment, and services. [This standard will not affect the accreditation decision at this time.]

Standard RC.02.01.01 The medical record contains information that reflects the patient's care, treatment, and services.

Standard RI.01.01.01 The hospital respects, protects, and promotes patient rights.

Standard RI.01.01.03 The hospital respects the patient's right to receive information in a manner he or she understands.

Standard HR.01.02.01 The hospital defines staff qualifications.

* **Source:** *2011 Comprehensive Accreditation Manual for Hospitals.* Please see the most current version of your organization's comprehensive accreditation manual for the most current standards and EPs.

In 2010 The Joint Commission published the monograph *Advancing Effective Communication, Cultural Competence, and Patient- and Family-Centered Care: A Roadmap for Hospitals* to help hospitals improve their communication with patients and family members. This monograph provides practice examples for improving communication with patients and family members at admission, assessment, treatment, transfer, and discharge. In addition, there are guidelines for improving communication with patients and family members when a patient transitions to end-of-life care. Finally, the monograph discusses the issues that leadership may face when working to improve communication between hospital staff and patients and provides practice exercises. The entire monograph can be accessed online at http://www.jointcommission.org/assets/1/6/ARoadmapforHospitalsfinalversion727.pdf.

Learning to communicate with and understand others in their field, whether verbally or in writing, presents a major challenge for many health care professionals. Their education and training have focused on subjects such as anatomy and chemistry or how to obtain a tissue sample, prepare and label a medication, read vital signs, and assess range of motion. Few have been taught how to talk to professionals from other disciplines collaboratively about a patient's needs and status. In recognition of the importance of effective communication in the delivery of care, interpersonal and communication skills are a required competency of medical residents under the Accreditation Council for Graduate Medical Education standards[30] and for maintenance of certification from the American Board of Medical Specialties.[31]

Hospitals that have committed to a culture of safety and quality will promote open communication between all levels and types of staff. Regular in-services on topics such as building a collaborative and safe corporate culture or working effectively as a health care team are a good starting point. It may also be helpful to train nurses, pharmacists, therapists, and others how to ask questions of physicians and one another. This instruction can include jargon or terms commonly used in the individual hospital or by different disciplines, methods of phrasing questions (and responses) in a nonconfrontational manner, and ways to verify unclear in-person or telephone communications.

Board members, senior managers, and other leaders who model good communication techniques further this endeavor. Authority figures who keep everyone in the hospital informed about important issues and deal with all staff in an open, nonthreatening manner set the stage for this type of interaction throughout the hospital.

Understanding Performance Improvement

The approaches to providing safe, high-quality care have gone through many incarnations in the past few decades—from the initial fault-finding of quality assurance, to the introduction of quantifiable measurement in continuous quality improvement, to the ongoing monitoring of important patient care and support functions under performance improvement. Performance improvement, a methodology for examining and improving processes and systems within a hospital, involves identifying an opportunity for improvement, collecting data on measures pertaining to the relevant process, analyzing those data, formulating a plan of action based on the results, implementing the plan, and monitoring the level of improvement through further data collection and analysis.

⊠ Standards in Practice ⊠

Established processes that focus on patient safety and quality are referred to in **Standard LD.03.03.01:** Leaders use hospitalwide planning to establish structures and processes that focus on safety and quality.*

* **Source:** *2011 Comprehensive Accreditation Manual for Hospitals.* Please see the most current version of your organization's comprehensive accreditation manual for the most current standards and EPs.

Performance measurement, a component of performance improvement, refers to the systematic collection of data over time (or at one point in time) and includes choosing measures, setting performance goals, evaluating and comparing data, planning and implementing data collection, and organizing and presenting data so the results can be used to improve processes. Performance measurement drives the data reports that board members receive about safety and quality issues such as falls, restraint use, or surgical site infections. However, it is imperative that data provided to board members be produced by highly reliable measurements. Inaccurate data collection could result in board members making decisions based on incorrect information.

To ensure highly reliable data collection and measurement, The Joint Commission recommends using Lean Thinking and Six Sigma, which are incorporated in RPI. (For more information on RPI, *see* page 5.)

Common Safety Areas of Concern

Each hospital must identify its own areas of vulnerability to risk, or areas of concern, based on the types and extent of services it offers and the patient populations it serves. However, some issues are fairly universal across a specific setting or across health care organizations. For example, hand-off communication is a common problem for hospitals, while staffing shortages, medication errors, infection control, and emergency management can be problematic for all settings along the continuum of care. All these issues are frequent topics of performance improvement activities and study.

Hand-off Communication

Hand-off communication—which occurs when patient care responsibilities are transferred from one health care worker to another—is a frequent and high-risk event. Researchers estimate that 80% of serious medical errors involve miscommunication between caregivers when patients are transferred, or handed off.[32] Although The Joint Commission has focused on hand-off communication since 2006, with the implementation of National Patient Safety Goal 2 for improving hand-off communication, organizations continue to struggle with standardizing a method for exchanging patient care information between the sending caregiver and the receiving caregiver.

To provide further assistance to organizations that struggle with hand-off communication, the Joint Commission Center for Transforming Healthcare has conducted a project with 10 leading hospitals to analyze barriers to effective hand-off communication and offer solutions, including the following[32]:

- ► Standardize the critical content (for example, patient history, treatment plan, key events).
- ► Hardwire your system by developing standardized forms, tools, or checklists to guide the discussion during hand-off communication.
- ► Allow opportunities to ask questions (and exchange contact information in the event that there are questions later).

- Collect and measure data to ensure the quality of hand-off communication.
- Educate and coach staff on what constitutes a successful handoff (education on hand-off communication should be standardized as well).

In 2011 the Center will be piloting targeted solutions for hand-off communication. Targeted solutions provide a step-by-step process for measuring performance, identifying barriers to excellent performance, and implementing solutions. Solutions that are proven to be effective will be added to the Targeted Solutions Tool, which is free for every accredited hospital. For up-to-date information on the hand-off communication tool, *see* http://www.centerfortransforminghealthcare.org/tst.aspx.

⊠ Standards in Practice ⊠

Improving hand-off communication and communication among caregivers is addressed in **National Patient Safety Goal 2**: Improve the effectiveness of communication among caregivers.*

* **Source:** *2011 Comprehensive Accreditation Manual for Hospitals.* Please see the most current version of your organization's comprehensive accreditation manual for the most current standards and EPs.

Staffing Shortages

To say that a great deal has been written about the current staffing crisis, particularly regarding nurses, would be an understatement. Effective staffing involves providing a sufficient number of appropriately skilled and competent staff to meet the needs of a hospital's patients. When a facility is well staffed, it is more likely to have better clinical outcomes, lower mortality rates, shorter lengths of stay, and reduced costs of care. Inadequate staffing takes an obvious toll on caregivers, often subjecting them to longer hours, heavier patient load, more paperwork, and more stress. There is also a significant risk to patient safety when existing staff are spread thin. An extensive body of research literature now strongly suggests that low nurse staffing increases the risk of poor patient outcomes in hospitals, such as medication errors, health care–associated infections, and patient falls.[33,34] Unfortunately, more and more hospitals are finding it difficult to supply the staff their patients require. More than 135,000 nursing positions in U.S. hospitals are unfilled, and the shortage of nurses may increase to 260,000 by 2025.[35] However, shortages are not limited to hospitals or the nursing profession. Long term care organizations, home health agencies, and ambulatory and behavioral health care facilities are also struggling with shortages of aides and assistants, pharmacists, technicians, and other staff.

Recruiting new staff with the appropriate skill mix is a challenging process, but the need to retain current staff is also a challenge—and one that is often overlooked. Health care organizations across the United States are implementing creative solutions, and many experts and panels are compiling success stories at regional and national levels.[36-38] Leaders and board members need to focus on building a collaborative, team-based culture that emphasizes mutual respect and high-quality communication among nurses, physicians, and other staff. Productivity and job satisfaction increase when people have a sense of ownership and empowerment in their jobs, which is a huge factor in retaining staff. Involving frontline staff in evaluating and simplifying processes to help prevent errors promotes this sense of empowerment; it is also practical because the people who know a process best are those who use it every day. Leaders need to perform regular reviews of staffing effectiveness so that any shortages can be addressed before they affect patient safety.[35]

Board members who want to explore useful strategies to address staffing challenges can review state and national reports, skim regional trade publications for updates on local developments, and look for opportunities to speak to colleagues locally and nationally about their experiences. Knowing what other hospitals are doing to reduce turnover, bolster the supply of labor, allocate staff effectively, and ensure patient safety can be important first steps.[33]

Medication Management

Medication errors top nearly every health care setting's list of problems. The process of medication management encompasses the key elements of selecting, procuring, storing, prescribing/ordering, preparing, dispensing, administering, and monitoring medications. Glitches are possible at any point in the process, from incomplete or illegible orders to inaccurate labeling to incorrect dosage. Several factors have made medication management increasingly difficult during the past few years[39]:

- ▶ The huge increase in the number of new drugs on the market
- ▶ The treatment of patients with comorbidities by several physicians who do

not communicate with each other about the medications they prescribe
- ▶ The use of mail-order pharmacies that provide neither personal communication with a pharmacist nor (in many cases) a double check of new medications against those already taken by the patient
- ▶ The overabundance of look-alike/sound-alike drugs that are used to treat very different conditions
- ▶ The use of herbal and other over-the-counter medications

The sharing of information can help hospitals identify possible causes and solutions for high-risk areas. The MEDMARX® system is a national online database that aggregates hospital medication error data and disseminates these data to participants. Hospitals that contribute to the database (all reports are anonymous and use a standardized format) can access information about common types of errors and find examples of how other hospitals have handled specific problems. MEDMARX allows users to review the causes and contributing factors associated with errors facilitywide, thereby identifying specific problem-prone systems or processes that may need improvement.[40]

One of the most problematic areas in medication management involves making sure that a hospital has an accurate list of a patient's current medications on admission and that the list is updated during treatment and given to the next care setting, provider, or practitioner. A hospital needs to adopt the process of medication reconciliation to obtain and document a complete list of each patient's home medications and to compare that list to the admission, transfer, or discharge orders.[41] Having such a process in place can help prevent errors by ensuring that required home medications are continued while in the health care facility, contraindicated home medications are discontinued, discrepancies in dosages or routines are resolved, and missed or duplicate doses are avoided.

Another important issue in medication management is the use of various types of technology, including computerized provider order entry, electronic medical records, computerized decision support systems, smart pumps, computerized notification about critical test results, computerized adverse drug event monitoring, bar-coding technology to assist with accurate medication administration, tools to help providers track abnormal test results, and automated dispensing machines. Making these and other tools available to staff can help improve communication, allow easier access to key drug information, provide calculation assistance for dosing, monitor patients' medication use for contraindications, and offer decision support to physicians in choosing medications. Most hospitals will likely want to implement many or all of these strategies but will not be able to afford to do so simultaneously. Ideally, the choice should be made on the basis of return on investment and ease of implementation, given the hospital's particular situation (for example, the vendor system used). Although few studies have published data about return on investment, research is ongoing and results are pending for several of these technologies.[42]

However, technology alone cannot prevent medication errors; the hospital must integrate that technology into existing care processes that focus on safety and quality. Health care organizations must understand the organizational and cultural changes commonly caused by implementation of major clinical information systems (particularly computerized provider order entry) and assess their readiness for these changes.[42] Leaders and staff must also assess the overall security of each technology and determine what changes in care processes will be required to make the best use of it. Finally, training must be planned and implemented to ensure that staff are comfortable with and knowledgeable about the new technology and can make suggestions for ways to use it to reduce errors.[39]

Infection Prevention and Control

The Centers for Disease Control and Prevention (CDC) estimates, using statistics from 2002, that 1.7 million health care–associated infections occur in hospitals each year, resulting in 99,000 associated deaths.[43] Adding these infections to the well-publicized outbreaks of H1N1 influenza in the United States and elsewhere, the increase in cases of HIV and hepatitis, the persistence of drug-resistant organisms such as vancomycin-resistant enterococci and methicillin-resistant *Staphylococcus aureus* (MRSA), and the fear of a bioterrorist use of anthrax or smallpox, it is no wonder that infection prevention and control is high on the list of concerns for most hospitals. Infection presents a serious threat to patients who are already frail and/or have weakened immune systems, such as infants, the elderly, those with cancer or AIDS, those in intensive care units, and those who have been rendered susceptible to infection by inappropriate use of antibiotics.[44] Therefore, an effective, well-integrated infection prevention and control plan is vital for any hospital.

An infection prevention and control plan involves surveillance (identifying risks of infection), prevention, control, and reporting. A hospital's program is ultimately concerned with reducing the risk of infection to patients, health care workers, and visitors, so its design must be based on the type and scope of care provided as well as the patient populations served. Because all areas of the hospital must be aware of and observe infection prevention and control practices, representatives from each area/department should be included in the design of the program. This is another situation in which the promotion of a culture of safety is essential because staff must be encouraged to actively look for and report infection issues.

Many types of health care–associated infections can result from ineffective infection prevention and control practices; some examples are surgical site infections, catheter-associated urinary tract infections, central venous catheter infections, ventilator-associated pneumonia, and communicable diseases associated with bacterial infection. System breakdowns can occur in areas such as hand hygiene practices, cleaning and disinfection of medical equipment, environmental safety, observance of universal precautions, and annual influenza vaccinations for health care staff. For example, the CDC recommends that all health care workers receive an annual influenza vaccination; however, fewer than half of workers report actually being immunized.[44] The Joint Commission also requires organizations to make influenza vaccines available to health care workers and licensed independent practitioners through Infection Prevention and Control (IC) Standard IC.02.04.01. Thus, a potential infection prevention and control plan for any organization would involve educating staff on such statistics as "Influenza outbreaks in hospitals and long-term care facilities have been attributed to low vaccination rates among health care professionals"[45] and other information in order to increase staff influenza vaccination rates. In addition, poor compliance with hand hygiene consistently affects most health care organizations even though it is one of the easiest and most important ways to prevent health care–associated infections. In an effort to increase hand hygiene compliance rates, the Joint Commission Center for Transforming Healthcare and eight of the country's leading health care organizations developed a Targeted Solutions Tool.[46] The Tool examines the specific reasons health care staff consistently fail to comply with hand hygiene practices, such as having their hands full or not being able to get to an inconveniently located sink, and then offers potential solutions that have been successful at other organizations.[46]

Emergency Management

Health care organizations must prepare for every kind of natural or man-made emergency. They need contingency plans for providing emergency care and procedures such as those for evacuation and decontamination. To develop a plan, the hospital needs to identify all emergencies that could occur within the facility and the community. Next, leaders and staff must decide how likely each possible event is and what effect it would have on the hospital and the community. This process allows leaders to prioritize the emergency management plan and concentrate resources on the most likely and potentially serious events. The plan can then be tailored according to these priorities.

Many factors must be considered in planning for any emergency situation, including maintaining internal and external lines of communication, finding room for a large influx of patients, maintaining supply inventories, calling in extra staff, and providing transportation and food for patients and staff. Emergency planning often focuses on hospital emergency departments and trauma centers, but in a communitywide emergency all health care organizations may be needed to help with triage and urgent care of victims, to shelter community members or patients who have been evacuated from other facilities, or to provide staff and/or supplies to other hospitals.

Health care organizations need to establish an "all-hazards command structure," also called an incident command system. This system goes into effect in an emergency to ensure an organized response as well as overall site management for the facility. It designates responsibilities and reporting relationships for leaders and staff members during the emergency and is usually divided into two branches: medical and administrative. For the system to work effectively, it should be adaptable to a wide variety of situations, clearly understood by everyone in the hospital, and integrated with the plans and systems of community response groups.

The Next Step

As you come to understand the various external and internal factors that influence your hospital's delivery of safe, high-quality care, you need to explore the goals and requirements of accreditation so that you can help improve and maintain that safety and quality. Chapter 2 provides an overview of The Joint Commission, its services, and its usefulness to health care organizations.

References

1. Kellis D.S.: Healthcare reform and the hospital industry: What can we expect? J *Healthc Manag* 55:283–296, Jul.–Aug. 2010.
2. Central Intelligence Agency: Country comparison: Infant mortality rate. *The World Factbook.* https://www.cia.gov/library/publications/the-world-factbook/rankorder/2091rank.html (accessed Dec. 1, 2010).
3. Centers for Disease Control and Prevention: Vital signs: Health insurance coverage and health care utilization—United States, 2006–2009 and January–March 2010. *Morbidity and Mortality Weekly Report* 59, Nov. 9, 2010. http://www.cdc.gov/mmwr/preview/mmwrhtml/mm59e1109a1.htm (accessed Dec. 1, 2010).
4. Mulvany C.: Healthcare reform: The good, the bad, and the transformational. *Healthc Financ Manage* 64:52–59, Jun. 2010.
5. Wallin V. Jr., Parrott L., Simon J.: Blunting the negative impact of healthcare reform. *Healthc Financ Manage* 64:62–66, Sep. 2010.
6. Society of Hospital Medicine (SHM): *Health Care Reform Implementation Timeline: Key Provisions Affecting Hospitalists.* Apr. 15, 2010. http://www.hospitalmedicine.org/AM/Template.cfm?Section=Advocacy_Policy& Template=/CM/ContentDisplay.cfm&ContentID=25521 (accessed Dec. 2, 2010).
7. Joint Commission Center for Transforming Healthcare: *About the Center: Facts about the Joint Commission Center for Transforming Healthcare.* http://www.centerfortransforminghealthcare.org/about/about.aspx (accessed Nov. 24, 2010).
8. President's Advisory Commission on Consumer Protection and Quality in the Health Care Industry: *Advisory Commission's Final Report.* Revised Jul. 18, 1998. http://www.hcqualitycommission.gov/final (accessed Sep. 10, 2010).
9. National Quality Forum: *Addressing National Priorities.* http://www.qualityforum.org/Setting_Priorities/Addressing_National_Priorities.aspx (accessed Nov. 27, 2010).
10. Medicare Payment Advisory Commission (MEDPAC): *Report to the Congress: Medicare Payment Policy.* http://medpac.gov/documents/Mar10_EntireReport.pdf (accessed Nov. 27, 2010).
11. Centers for Medicare & Medicaid Services (CMS): *Hospital-Acquired Conditions.* http://www.cms.gov/HospitalAcqCond/06_Hospital-Acquired_Conditions.asp#TopOfPage (accessed Nov. 25, 2010).
12. Institute of Medicine: *To Err Is Human: Building a Safer Health System.* Washington, DC: National Academy Press, 1999.
13. Institute of Medicine: *Crossing the Quality Chasm: A New Health System for the 21st Century.* Washington, DC: National Academy Press, 2001.
14. Berwick D.M.: A user's manual for the IOM's "Quality Chasm" report. *Health Aff (Millwood)* 21:80–90, May–Jun. 2002.
15. The Leapfrog Group: *The Leapfrog Group Fact Sheet.* http://www.leapfroggroup.org/about_us/leapfrog-factsheet (accessed Sep. 10, 2010).
16. Institute for Healthcare Improvement: *Protecting 5 Million Lives from Harm.* http://www.ihi.org/IHI/Programs/Campaign/Campaign.htm?TabId=0 (accessed Sep. 10, 2010).
17. National Academy for State Health Policy: *Patient Safety Toolbox.* http://www.nashp.org/pst-welcome (accessed Nov. 27, 2010).
18. Association for Professionals in Infection Control and Epidemiology: *Legislation in Progress.* http://www.apic.org/map/index.htm (accessed Sep. 10, 2010).

19. Nelson E.C., et al.: Publicly reporting comprehensive quality and cost data: A health care system's transparency initiative. *Jt Comm J Qual Patient Saf* 31:573–584, Oct. 2005.
20. Orlikoff J.E., Totten M.: Governance in the spotlight: What the Sarbanes-Oxley Act means for you. *Trustee* 57:15–18, Sep. 2004.
21. Barr P.: Setting a good example. *Mod Healthc* 34:6–7, 14–15, Dec. 6, 2004.
22. Greene J.: Looking harder: The audit committee under Sarbanes-Oxley. *Trustee* 58:10–12, Jan. 2005.
23. Mantone J.: States turn up the heat. *Mod Healthc* 36:6–7, 16, Jan. 30, 2006.
24. Entwistle V.A., Mello M.M., Brennan T.A.: Advising patients about patient safety: Current initiatives risk shifting responsibility. *Jt Comm J Qual Patient Saf* 31:483–494, Sep. 2005.
25. Agency for Healthcare Research and Quality: *20 Tips to Help Prevent Medical Errors,* Feb. 2000. http://www.ahrq.gov/consumer/20tips.htm (accessed Sep. 10, 2010).
26. The Joint Commission: *Speak Up: Help Prevent Errors in Your Care.* http://www.jointcommission.org/speak_up_help_prevent_errors_in_your_care/ (accessed Mar. 3, 2011).
27. Roizen M.F., Oz M.C., Joint Commission: *YOU: The Smart Patient: An Insider's Handbook for Getting the Best Treatment.* New York: The Free Press, 2006.
28. The Joint Commission: *Summary Data of Sentinel Events Reviewed by The Joint Commission.* http://www.jointcommission.org/sentinel_event_statistics_quarterly/ (accessed Mar. 3, 2011).
29. Cohen M.M., et al.: Implementing a hospitalwide patient safety program for cultural change. In Frankel A.S. (ed.): *Strategies for Building a Hospitalwide Culture of Safety.* Oakbrook Terrace, IL: Joint Commission Resources, 2006, pp. 83–90.
30. Accreditation Council for Graduate Medical Education: *Common Program Requirements: General Competencies.* http://www.acgme.org/outcome/comp/GeneralCompetenciesStandards21307.pdf (accessed Sep. 10, 2010).
31. Nahrwold D.: The changing role of certification for physicians. *ABMS Reporter* 11, Spring 2002.
32. Joint Commission Center for Transforming Healthcare: *Facts about Hand-off Communications.* http://www.centerfortransforminghealthcare.org/projects/about_handoff_communication.aspx?print=y (accessed Nov. 27, 2010).
33. Clarke S.: Staffing the organization for excellence. In *From Front Office to Front Line: Essential Issues for Health Care Leaders.* Oakbrook Terrace, IL: Joint Commission Resources, 2005, pp. 113–144.
34. Rogers A.E., et al.: The working hours of hospital staff nurses and patient safety. *Health Aff (Millwood)* 23:202–212, Jul.–Aug. 2004.
35. American Association of Colleges of Nursing: *Nursing Shortage: Fact Sheet.* Updated Sep. 20, 2010. http://www.aacn.nche.edu/media/FactSheets/NursingShortage.htm (accessed Feb. 27, 2011).
36. American Hospital Association (AHA) Commission on Workforce for Hospitals and Health Systems: *In Our Hands: How Hospital Leaders Can Build a Thriving Workforce.* Chicago: AHA, Apr. 2002.
37. Pennsylvania Department of Health: *State Health Improvement Plan: White Paper: The Nurse Workforce in Pennsylvania.* Harrisburg, PA: Pennsylvania Department of Health, Jun. 2004.
38. The Joint Commission: *Health Care at the Crossroads: Strategies for Addressing the Evolving Nursing Crisis.* Oakbrook Terrace, IL: Joint Commission Resources, 2002.
39. The Joint Commission: *Using Technology to Improve Medication Safety.* Oakbrook Terrace, IL: Joint Commission Resources, 2005.
40. Santell J.P.: Medication errors: Experience of the United States Pharmacopeia (USP). *Jt Comm J Qual Patient Saf* 31:114–119, Feb. 2005.

41. Tips for reconciling medications across the continuum. *Joint Commission: The Source* 3:3–4, Apr. 2005.
42. Kuperman G.J., Bates D.W.: Using information technology to improve health care safety and quality. In *From Front Office to Front Line: Essential Issues for Health Care Leaders.* Oakbrook Terrace, IL: Joint Commission Resources, 2005, pp. 65–89.
43. Centers for Disease Control and Prevention (CDC): *Healthcare-Associated Infections (HAIs).* http://www.cdc.gov/HAI/burden.html (accessed Feb. 27, 2011).
44. The Joint Commission: *The Joint Commission Guide to Priority Focus Areas.* Oakbrook Terrace, IL: Joint Commission Resources, 2004.
45. Centers for Disease Control and Prevention (CDC): *Influenza Vaccination Information for Health Care Workers.* http://www.cdc.gov/flu/HealthcareWorkers.htm (accessed Nov. 23, 2010).
46. Joint Commission Center for Transforming Healthcare: *Facts about the Hand Hygiene Project.* http://www.centerfortransforminghealthcare.org/projects/about_hand_hygiene_project.aspx (accessed Nov. 24, 2010).

Chapter 2

What You Need to Know About The Joint Commission

As a hospital board member, you may be most familiar with The Joint Commission as an accrediting body, but it has many other aspects that also can be useful to your organization as you work to improve quality and safety. This chapter provides an overview of the Joint Commission's work in accreditation, performance measurement, patient safety, information dissemination, and public policy initiatives. Established in 1951, The Joint Commission (known until January 2007 as the Joint Commission on Accreditation of Healthcare Organizations) offers many services geared toward fulfilling its basic vision of improving the safety and quality of care provided by health care organizations. The Joint Commission enterprise actually consists of several entities with complementary missions. Accreditation, certification, standards development, and performance measurement are handled through The Joint Commission. Consultative services, educational programs, books and periodicals, and electronic learning products are provided by Joint Commission Resources (JCR), a not-for-profit affiliate of The Joint Commission. A component of JCR— Joint Commission International (JCI)—provides international accreditation, consultation, and education to improve the quality of care and patient safety. To date, 300 public and private health care organizations in 39 countries are accredited by JCI. Established in 2009, the Joint Commission Center for Transforming Healthcare aims to solve health care's most critical safety and quality problems. The Center's participants—the nation's leading hospitals and health systems—use a systematic approach to analyze specific breakdowns in care, discover their underlying causes, and develop targeted solutions for these complex problems.

Accreditation, Certification, Standards, and Measures

More than 18,000 health care providers in the United States use Joint Commission standards and performance measures to guide how they administer care and continuously improve performance. Accreditation is provided for the following types of organizations:

- General, psychiatric, children's, and rehabilitation hospitals
- Critical access hospitals
- Medical equipment services, hospice services, home care pharmacy, and other home care organizations
- Nursing homes and other long term care facilities
- Behavioral health care organizations, addiction services, and foster care
- Rehabilitation centers, group practices, office-based surgery organizations, and other ambulatory care providers
- Independent or freestanding laboratories

The Joint Commission also provides certification in disease-specific care and health care staffing services. The disease-specific care program and standards can be applied to hospitals, ambulatory care, long term care, home care, behavioral health care, and disease management service companies. The Joint Commission has advanced certification programs for heart failure, chronic kidney disease, chronic obstructive pulmonary disease, inpatient diabetes care, primary stroke, lung volume reduction surgery, and ventricular assist devices for destination therapy. The disease-specific care program's model can be applied to the management of almost any chronic disease or condition; examples of programs that have been certified include those for the following:

- Alzheimer's disease
- Arthritis
- Asthma
- Cancer
- Chronic obstructive pulmonary disease
- Congestive heart failure
- Coronary artery disease
- Depression
- Emphysema

- Epilepsy
- High-risk pregnancy
- HIV/AIDS
- Hypertension
- Multiple sclerosis
- Obesity/bariatric surgery

Each program is evaluated for its ability to integrate and coordinate care based on sound chronic care management principles.

To be eligible to receive payments from Medicare—the federal program that provides health care benefits to more than 42 million elderly and disabled beneficiaries—hospitals must meet certain criteria established by federal law. The Centers for Medicare & Medicaid Services (CMS), the federal agency within the U.S. Department of Health & Human Services that administers Medicare, has established Conditions of Participation that hospitals must meet to be eligible to participate in the Medicare program. Hospitals that meet the Joint Commission's accreditation standards are deemed eligible for Medicare payment.

Accreditation and certification are also important because thorough and ongoing evaluation of processes and performance is the cornerstone of continuous improvement. The Joint Commission publishes standards for each type of organization it accredits or certifies. These standards address the performance of key functions within the organization and define the performance expectations, structures, and processes necessary to ensure safe, high-quality care. Nearly all of the standards directly address safety concerns such as infection prevention and control, medication management, staffing and staff competency, fire safety, security, restraint and seclusion, emergency management, and surgery and anesthesia. The Joint Commission develops its standards in consultation with health care experts, providers, measurement experts, purchasers, and consumers. Specific issues include the following:

- Implementing a patient safety program
- Responding to adverse events
- Proactively analyzing and redesigning systems to prevent harm
- Communicating all outcomes of care (positive or negative) to patients

The governing body's responsibilities are included in the Leadership standards (LD) for each accreditation program (*see* Sidebar 2-1 on pages 37–44). The Joint Commission revised the Leadership standards in 2009 to help the governing body, chief executive officer, leaders of the medical staff, and other executives to work collaboratively. Together, the leaders of the organization create a culture of safety by promoting trust and fairness and encouraging staff to report risks and adverse events. The governing body's responsibilities include the following:

- *Mission and strategic planning.* This includes an examination of community needs to define the organization's role and purpose; an assessment of the organization's capabilities; development and support of the organization's mission, vision, and values; and strategic planning for the future.
- *Quality of care and patient safety.* Board members must ensure that performance improvement and patient safety programs are implemented, that effective processes exist and are followed for credentialing and privileging, and that risk management is carried out.
- *Leadership.* This includes ensuring effective management through an established process of selecting a chief executive officer, meeting legal and accreditation requirements, resolving conflict among leaders, and empowering leaders across the organization.
- *Budget and finance.* Boards must provide the necessary resources for patient care, patient safety, staffing, and performance improvement.
- *Board effectiveness.* A governing body is responsible for assessing and improving its own conduct. This means establishing policies and procedures for the board, understanding its role in organizational leadership, evaluating its ability to carry out its duties, and seeking new members (if applicable).

The Joint Commission's accreditation process has undergone significant changes since 2004. Shifting its direction from survey preparation to continuous improvement, the process focuses on systems that are critical to patient safety and quality of care. It encourages organizations to use the standards as guidelines for day-to-day oversight of operations, and standards have been revised and streamlined for this purpose. A more detailed explanation of the accreditation process is provided in your accreditation manual; this section highlights some of the key features with which you should be familiar.

Sidebar 2-1. Joint Commission Leadership Requirements Relevant to Governing Body Members*

Standard LD.01.01.01
The hospital has a leadership structure.

Rationale for LD.01.01.01
Every hospital has a leadership structure to support operations and the provision of care. In many hospitals this structure is formed by three leadership groups: the governing body, senior managers, and the organized medical staff. In some hospitals there may be two leadership groups, and in others only one. Individual leaders may participate in more than one group.

Elements of Performance for LD.01.01.01
▲ 1. The hospital identifies those responsible for governance.
▲ 2. The governing body identifies those responsible for planning, management, and operational activities.
▲ 3. The governing body identifies those responsible for the provision of care, treatment, and services.

Standard LD.01.02.01
The hospital identifies the responsibilities of its leaders.

Rationale for LD.01.02.01
Many responsibilities may be shared by all leaders. Others are assigned by the governing body to senior managers and the leaders of the organized medical staff. Hospital performance depends on how well the leaders work together to carry out these responsibilities.

Elements of Performance for LD.01.02.01
▲ 1. Senior managers and leaders of the organized medical staff work with the governing body to define their shared and unique responsibilities and accountabilities.
▲ 2. The governing body establishes a process for making decisions when a leadership group fails to fulfill its responsibilities and/or accountabilities.

(continued on page 38)

---
* Although every standard in the "Leadership" (LD) chapter applies to board members, the standards highlighted in this box focus attention on these leadership requirements.

> **Sidebar 2-1. Joint Commission Leadership Requirements Relevant to Governing Body Members (continued)**
>
> **C 4. For hospitals that use Joint Commission accreditation for deemed status purposes:** The chief executive officer, medical staff, and nurse executive make certain that hospitalwide performance improvement and training programs address problems identified by the individual responsible for infection prevention and control and that corrective action plans are successfully implemented.
>
> **Standard LD.01.03.01**
> The governing body is ultimately accountable for the safety and quality of care, treatment, and services.
>
> **Rationale for LD.01.03.01**
> The governing body's ultimate responsibility for safety and quality derives from its legal responsibility and operational authority for hospital performance. In this context, the governing body provides for internal structures and resources (including staff) that support safety and quality.
>
> **Elements of Performance for LD.01.03.01**
> **A** 1. The governing body defines in writing its responsibilities.
> **A** 2. The governing body provides for organization management and planning.
> **A** 3. The governing body approves the hospital's written scope of services.
>   **Note:** *For hospitals that use Joint Commission accreditation for deemed status purposes:* If emergency services are provided at the hospital, the hospital complies with the requirements of 42 CFR 482.55. For more information on 42 CFR 482.55, refer to the "Medicare Requirements for Hospitals" appendix.
> **A** 4. The governing body selects the chief executive responsible for managing the hospital.
> **A** 5. The governing body provides for the resources needed to maintain safe, quality care, treatment, and services.
> **A** 6. The governing body works with the senior managers and leaders of the organized medical staff to annually evaluate the hospital's performance in relation to its mission, vision, and goals.
> **A** 7. The governing body provides a system for resolving conflicts among individuals working in the hospital.
>
> *(continued on page 39)*

Sidebar 2-1. Joint Commission Leadership Requirements Relevant to Governing Body Members (continued)

A 8. The governing body provides the organized medical staff with the opportunity to participate in governance.

A 9. The governing body provides the organized medical staff with the opportunity to be represented at governing body meetings (through attendance and voice) by one or more of its members, as selected by the organized medical staff.

A 10. Organized medical staff members are eligible for full membership in the hospital's governing body, unless legally prohibited.

Standard LD.01.07.01

The governing body, senior managers, and leaders of the organized medical staff have the knowledge needed for their roles in the hospital, or they seek guidance to fulfill their roles.

Elements of Performance for LD.01.07.01

A 1. The governing body, senior managers, and leaders of the organized medical staff work together to identify the skills required of individual leaders.

C 2. Individual members of the governing body, senior managers, and leaders of the organized medical staff are oriented to all of the following:
- The hospital's mission and vision
- The hospital's safety and quality goals
- The hospital's structure and the decision-making process
- The development of the budget as well as the interpretation of the hospital's financial statements
- The population(s) served by the hospital and any issues related to that population(s)
- The individual and interdependent responsibilities and accountabilities of the governing body, senior managers, and leaders of organized medical staff as they relate to supporting the mission of the hospital and to providing safe and quality care
- Applicable law and regulation

A 3. The governing body provides leaders with access to information and training in areas where they need additional skills or expertise.

(continued on page 40)

Sidebar 2-1. Joint Commission Leadership Requirements Relevant to Governing Body Members (continued)

Standard LD.02.02.01
The governing body, senior managers, and leaders of the organized medical staff address any conflict of interest involving leaders that affect or could affect the safety or quality of care, treatment, and services.
Note: *This standard addresses conflict of interest involving individual members of leadership groups. For conflicts of interest among staff and licensed independent practitioners who are not members of leadership groups, see* Standard LD.04.02.01.

Rationale for LD.02.02.01
Conflicts of interest can occur in many circumstances and may involve professional or business relationships. Leaders create policies that provide for the oversight and control of these situations. Together, leaders address actual and potential conflicts of interest that could interfere with the hospital's responsibility to the community it serves.

Elements of Performance for LD.02.02.01
▲ 1. The governing body, senior managers, and leaders of the organized medical staff work together to define, in writing, conflicts of interest involving leaders that could affect safety and quality of care, treatment, and services.
▲ 2. The governing body, senior managers, and leaders of the organized medical staff work together to develop a written policy that defines how conflicts of interest involving leaders will be addressed.
▲ 3. Conflicts of interest involving leaders are disclosed as defined by the hospital.

Standard LD.02.03.01
The governing body, senior managers, and leaders of the organized medical staff regularly communicate with each other on issues of safety and quality.

Rationale for LD.02.03.01
Leaders, who provide for safety and quality, must communicate with each other on matters affecting the hospital and those it serves. The safety and quality of care, treatment, and services depend on open communication. Civility among leaders fosters such communication. Ideally, this will result in trust and mutual respect among those who work in the hospital.

(continued on page 41)

Sidebar 2-1. Joint Commission Leadership Requirements Relevant to Governing Body Members (continued)

Elements of Performance for LD.02.03.01
- **A** 1. Leaders discuss issues that affect the hospital and the population(s) it serves, including the following:
  - Performance improvement activities
  - Reported safety and quality issues
  - Proposed solutions and their impact on the hospital's resources
  - Reports on key quality measures and safety indicators
  - Safety and quality issues specific to the population(s) served
  - Input from the population(s) served
- **A** 2. The hospital establishes time frames for the discussion of issues that affect the hospital and the population(s) it serves.

Standard LD.02.04.01
The hospital manages conflict between leadership groups to protect the quality and safety of care.

Elements of Performance for LD.02.04.01
- **A** 1. Senior managers and leaders of the organized medical staff work with the governing body to develop an ongoing process for managing conflict among leadership groups.
- **A** 2. The governing body approves the process for managing conflict among leadership groups.
- **A** 4. The conflict management process includes the following:
  - Meeting with the involved parties as early as possible to identify the conflict
  - Gathering information regarding the conflict
  - Working with the parties to manage and, when possible, resolve the conflict
  - Protecting the safety and quality of care
- **A** 5. The hospital implements the process when a conflict arises that, if not managed, could adversely affect patient safety or quality of care.

Standard LD.03.01.01
Leaders create and maintain a culture of safety and quality throughout the hospital.

(continued on page 42)

Sidebar 2-1. Joint Commission Leadership Requirements Relevant to Governing Body Members (continued)

Elements of Performance for LD.03.01.01
- A 1. Leaders regularly evaluate the culture of safety and quality using valid and reliable tools.
- A 2. Leaders prioritize and implement changes identified by the evaluation.
- A 3. Leaders provide opportunities for all individuals who work in the hospital to participate in safety and quality initiatives.
- A 4. Leaders develop a code of conduct that defines acceptable, disruptive, and inappropriate behaviors.
- A 5. Leaders create and implement a process for managing disruptive and inappropriate behaviors.
- A 6. Leaders provide education that focuses on safety and quality for all individuals.
- A 7. Leaders establish a team approach among all staff at all levels.
- A 8. All individuals who work in the hospital, including staff and licensed independent practitioners, are able to openly discuss issues of safety and quality. (See also LD.04.04.05, EP 6)
- A 9. Literature and advisories relevant to patient safety are available to all individuals who work in the hospital.
- A 10. Leaders define how members of the population(s) served can help identify and manage issues of safety and quality within the hospital.

Standard LD.03.02.01
The hospital uses data and information to guide decisions and to understand variation in the performance of processes supporting safety and quality.

Elements of Performance for LD.03.02.01
- A 1. Leaders set expectations for using data and information to improve the safety and quality of care, treatment, and services.
- A 3. The hospital uses processes to support systematic data and information use.
- A 4. Leaders provide the resources needed for data and information use, including staff, equipment, and information systems.
- A 5. The hospital uses data and information in decision making that supports the safety and quality of care, treatment, and services. (See also NR.02.01.01, EPs 3 and 6; PI.02.01.01, EP 8)

(continued on page 43)

Sidebar 2-1. Joint Commission Leadership Requirements Relevant to Governing Body Members (continued)

▲ 6. The hospital uses data and information to identify and respond to internal and external changes in the environment.
▲ 7. Leaders evaluate how effectively data and information are used throughout the hospital.

Standard LD.03.03.01
Leaders use hospitalwide planning to establish structures and processes that focus on safety and quality.

Elements of Performance for LD.03.03.01
▲ 1. Planning activities focus on improving patient safety and health care quality.
▲ 3. Planning is systematic, and it involves designated individuals and information sources.
▲ 4. Leaders provide the resources needed to support the safety and quality of care, treatment, and services.
▲ 5. Safety and quality planning is hospitalwide.
▲ 6. Planning activities adapt to changes in the environment.
▲ 7. Leaders evaluate the effectiveness of planning activities.

Standard LD.03.04.01
The hospital communicates information related to safety and quality to those who need it, including staff, licensed independent practitioners, patients, families, and external interested parties.

Elements of Performance for LD.03.04.01
▲ 1. Communication processes foster the safety of the patient and the quality of care.
▲ 3. Communication is designed to meet the needs of internal and external users.
▲ 4. Leaders provide the resources required for communication, based on the needs of patients, the community, physicians, staff, and management.
▲ 5. Communication supports safety and quality throughout the hospital. (*See also* LD.04.04.05, EPs 6 and 12)
▲ 6. When changes in the environment occur, the hospital communicates those changes effectively.
▲ 7. Leaders evaluate the effectiveness of communication methods.

(continued on page 44)

Sidebar 2-1. Joint Commission Leadership Requirements Relevant to Governing Body Members (continued)

Standard LD.03.05.01
Leaders implement changes in existing processes to improve the performance of the hospital.

Elements of Performance for LD.03.05.01
- **A** 1. Structures for managing change and performance improvements exist that foster the safety of the patient and the quality of care, treatment, and services.
- **A** 3. The hospital has a systematic approach to change and performance improvement.
- **A** 4. Leaders provide the resources required for performance improvement and change management, including sufficient staff, access to information, and training.
- **A** 5. The management of change and performance improvement supports both safety and quality throughout the hospital.
- **A** 6. The hospital's internal structures can adapt to changes in the environment.
- **A** 7. Leaders evaluate the effectiveness of processes for the management of change and performance improvement. (See also PI.02.01.01, EP 13)

Standard LD.03.06.01
Those who work in the hospital are focused on improving safety and quality.

Elements of Performance for LD.03.06.01
- **A** 1. Leaders design work processes to focus individuals on safety and quality issues.
- **A** 3. Leaders provide for a sufficient number and mix of individuals to support safe, quality care, treatment, and services.
  Note: *The number and mix of individuals is appropriate to the scope and complexity of the services offered.*
- **A** 4. Those who work in the hospital are competent to complete their assigned responsibilities.
- **A** 5. Those who work in the hospital adapt to changes in the environment.
- **A** 6. Leaders evaluate the effectiveness of those who work in the hospital to promote safety and quality.

Priority Focus Process

The Priority Focus Process is a data-driven methodology that consistently uses presurvey information about health care organizations to create priorities for reviewing standards compliance, thus lending consistency to the survey process. Presurvey information is gathered from an organization's application for accreditation, the organization's past survey findings, the Joint Commission's Quality Monitoring System database of complaints and non–self-reported sentinel events, any ORYX® core performance measure data, and certain external data, if available. External data consist of publicly available data that are applicable to the accreditation program(s) being surveyed, such as the *Hospital Consumer Assessment of Healthcare Providers and Systems.*

The Joint Commission integrates the data and uses them to identify the top four or five relevant priority focus areas and clinical/service groups applicable to the organization. Priority focus areas are processes, systems, and structures in a health care organization that significantly affect safety and/or the quality of care. A list of the priority focus areas for hospitals is provided in Table 2-1 below. Clinical/service groups define patient populations and/or services provided by the organization (*see* Table 2-2, page 46 for a list of hospital clinical/service groups). The lists of priority focus areas and clinical/service groups identify potential risk points in areas that are especially relevant to providing safe, high-quality care to patients in your particular organization.

Table 2-1. Priority Focus Areas

- Assessment & Care/Services
- Communication
- Credentialed Practitioners
- Equipment Use
- Infection Control
- Information Management
- Medication Management
- Organizational Structure
- Orientation and Training
- Patient Safety
- Physical Environment
- Quality Improvement Expertise/Activities
- Rights & Ethics
- Staffing

Table 2-2. Hospital Clinical/Service Groups

- Cardiac surgery
- Cardiology (ORYX® core measure area)
- Dentistry
- Dermatology
- Endocrinology
- Gastroenterology
- General medicine
- General surgery
- Gynecology
- Hematology
- HIV infection
- Neonatology (ORYX core measure area)
- Nephrology
- Neurology
- Neurosurgery
- Normal newborns
- Obstetrics (ORYX core measure area)
- Oncology
- Ophthalmology
- Orthopedics
- Otolaryngology
- Pediatrics (ORYX core measure area)
- Psychiatry
- Pulmonary (ORYX core measure area)
- Rehabilitation
- Rheumatology
- Substance abuse
- Thoracic surgery
- Trauma
- Urology
- Vascular surgery
- Other

This data and information become the basis for Priority Focus Process Reports. The reports, updated quarterly, pull in data up to three years prior to the date The Joint Commission runs the tool (laboratories pull in data for the previous two years). Accredited organizations are automatically notified when an updated report is available on their secure *Joint Commission Connect*™ extranet site. The report also is made available to Joint Commission surveyors prior to conducting an on-site survey.

Surveyors use the identified priority focus areas and clinical/service groups (along with other organization-specific data) to develop a better understanding of the hospital's systems and processes and the patient services it provides. This information helps surveyors develop the initial structure of the survey by identifying relevant standards to be addressed on site as well as patient populations that should be represented in tracer activities (described later in this chapter). Based on initial findings, surveyors may broaden or change the focus of the on-site survey as appropriate.

✪ Trustees Taking the Lead ✪

Remember that the list of priority focus areas and clinical/service groups identifies potential risks in areas that are especially important to providing safe, high-quality care to patients in your particular organization. To help evaluate the current level of safety and quality of care, you can encourage management and staff to conduct self-audits and mock tracers based on their top clinical/service groups and priority focus areas.

Unannounced Surveys

Since January 2006, The Joint Commission has been conducting unannounced surveys of accredited organizations. This survey process emphasizes the tenet that safe, high-quality care should be provided at all times and that organizations should not have to "ramp up" for an on-site survey. Staff members focus on their everyday processes rather than on making quick fixes to comply with standards just before a survey, and surveyors are able to observe care being provided under normal circumstances. The shift to unannounced surveys also provides accountability and raises the degree of confidence the public can have in accredited health care providers. If an organization has truly incorporated the standards into its systems, it will be in compliance no matter when the survey is conducted, and the public will be assured that safe, high-quality care is provided all the time.

✪ Trustees Taking the Lead ✪

Although administrative staff may keep board members updated on how well their organization is complying with Joint Commission requirements, it is important that board members take advantage of their own opportunities to participate in various stages of the accreditation process. For example, some board members may want to meet with surveyors during on-site surveys.

A board presence at any type of evaluative meeting—whether it is an accreditation survey, a public health survey, or an interview with an award committee—shows that the entire organization is involved in and committed to providing high-quality care. Therefore, board members should charge management with apprising them of these opportunities and allowing them to participate and contribute.

Table 2-3. Exceptions to Unannounced Surveys

Subject	Exception
Initial surveys	Announced (unless deemed status requirements specify unannounced surveys)
Early Survey Policy—1st and 2nd survey	Announced (unless deemed status requirements specify unannounced surveys)
Organization undergoing Periodic Performance Review option 2 and option 3 surveys	7-day notice
Department of Defense facilities	7 days within certain periods of time

The Joint Commission generally conducts surveys unannounced except when it would not be logical or feasible. Table 2-3, above, outlines specific exceptions to unannounced surveys and the length of advance notice.

Tracer Methodology

An important component of the on-site survey process is tracer methodology, which assesses care, treatment, and services by following the actual experiences of patients within the different areas of the health care organization. There are three types of tracers:

1. Program-specific tracers
2. Individual tracers
3. System tracers

The goal of the program-specific tracer is to identify safety concerns within different levels and types of care, treatment, or services. Program-specific tracers focus on important issues relevant to types of care, treatment, or services offered by the organization; programs being surveyed; and the organization's priority focus areas.

In an individual tracer activity, the surveyor uses the organization's priority focus information to identify specific patients and follow the care of those patients from admission through discharge or transfer. (For laboratories, patient samples are traced from physician order through notification and documentation.) Surveyors try to select patients who are in the organization's top clinical/service groups, who cross programs and/or have received care in multiple areas (such as a nursing home resident who is admitted to a hospital and then transferred to a rehabilitation facility), and who have been in contact with areas related to the individual-based system topics (infection control, medication management, and data use). Viewing the organization's systems from the patient's perspective allows an evaluation of both the components of a system and how the different systems work together as a whole.

A system tracer focuses on a specific system or process across the entire organization. The surveyor uses information obtained from individual tracers and discussions with staff members to trace one or more of the following systems:

- *Data use,* which looks at how the organization collects, analyzes, and interprets data to improve patient safety and care
- *Infection control,* which focuses on the organization's processes for the prevention, control, and surveillance of infection
- *Medication management,* which explores the organization's medication processes and subprocesses from procurement to monitoring of effects, as well as at potential risk points

Because errors are so prevalent when patients are handed off between programs, units, organizations, and individual practitioners, surveyors pay particular attention to how staff and processes interact and coordinate care at transitions.

Performance Measurement and the ORYX® Initiative

One of the ways that performance measurement data are integrated into the accreditation process is through the ORYX initiative, which began in 1997 and has evolved in recent years. A key component of ORYX is the identification and use of core measures—standardized performance measures for specific conditions and populations with precisely defined data elements, calculation algorithms, and consistent data collection protocols. These measures are grouped into sets; approved core measure sets cover the following conditions:

- Acute myocardial infarction
- Heart failure
- Pneumonia

- Surgical Care Improvement Project
- Hospital outpatient department
- Children's asthma care
- Stroke
- Venous thromboembolism
- Hospital-based inpatient psychiatric services
- Perinatal care

Future measure sets are anticipated to include tobacco and alcohol measures, patient blood management, and nursing-sensitive care.

Since 2004 The Joint Commission and CMS have been working together to align measures common to both organizations. These standardized common measures, called National Hospital Inpatient Quality Measures, are integral to improving the quality of care provided to hospital patients and bringing value to stakeholders by focusing on the actual results of care. Measure alignment benefits hospitals by making it easier and less costly to collect and report data because the same data set can be used to satisfy both CMS and Joint Commission requirements. All of the National Hospital Inpatient Quality Measures common to The Joint Commission and CMS are endorsed by the National Quality Forum. Detailed information on core measures can be found on the Joint Commission's Web site at http://www.jointcommission.org/performance_measurement.aspx.

General ORYX Requirements for Hospitals

Hospitals must collect and transmit data to The Joint Commission on a minimum of four core measure sets or, depending on the number of applicable core measure sets available, a combination of core measure sets and up to nine non-core measures.

With the exception of Joint Commission–accredited children's hospitals that are required to use the children's asthma care core measure set and freestanding psychiatric hospitals that are required to use the hospital-based inpatient psychiatric services core measure set, the selection of core measure sets is at the discretion of the hospital. Data for all applicable measures must be submitted through performance measurement system vendors that have been evaluated and listed by The Joint Commission.

Vendors submit aggregate monthly hospital data on a quarterly basis to The Joint Commission. Following each submission of quarterly data, The Joint Commission generates an ORYX Performance Measurement Report and posts it on each hospital's secure *Joint Commission Connect* extranet site. Board members often receive these summary reports or highlights from the hospital administration as part of regular improvement data reports. The report provides the hospital with a summary analysis of its performance at the measure set level and for each individual measure. Through the use of control charts and "target" charts created for each measure, the hospital gets information on the stability over time of the process addressed by each measure along with an analysis of the hospital's performance against a measure target rate based on the national rate of performance on each core measure. At the time of survey, poor performance against the national target for a specific measure for three of the most recent four quarters will require the hospital to provide the surveyor with evidence of a credible analysis of its outlier status on the measure. Participation in ORYX and the use of core measures is mandatory for Joint Commission–accredited hospitals.

Accountability Measures

The Joint Commission has categorized its performance measures into accountability and non-accountability measures in an effort to promote excellence in the delivery of care and maximize health outcomes as well as in anticipation of the CMS incentive payments that become effective in 2013. Accountability measures meet the four criteria that produce the greatest positive impact on patient outcomes as demonstrated by hospitals:

1. **Research:** Strong scientific evidence demonstrates that compliance with the process of care improves health care outcomes.
2. **Proximity:** The process being measured is closely connected to the outcome it impacts.
3. **Accuracy:** The measure can judge whether the process has been delivered with sufficient effectiveness to make improved outcomes likely.
4. **Adverse Effects:** The measure is designed to minimize or eliminate unintended adverse events.

Examples of accountability measures include giving aspirin to heart attack patients upon both arrival and discharge, vaccinating pneumonia patients against influenza, and administering antibiotics within one hour before patients get their first surgical cut. On the other hand, non-accountability measures provide good advice in providing appropriate patient care. Examples of non-accountability measures include smoking cessation counseling, administration of antibiotics within six hours of arrival for patients diagnosed with pneumonia, and left ventricular systolic function assessment for patients diagnosed with heart failure.

Accountability measures have been integrated into the information reported on the Joint Commission's Quality Check® Web site (only accountability measures are used to calculate the overall performance rate for each measure set) and the Priority Focus Process (accountability measures are more heavily weighted). In the future, The Joint Commission will eliminate measures that do not work well, incorporate performance on accountability measures in accreditation standards, and include only accountability measures in the ORYX program.

Library of Other Measures

In March 2010 The Joint Commission established a library of performance improvement measures, which provides health care organizations and other stakeholders with ready access to reliable, tested, and evidence-based measures that can be used to improve the safety and quality of health care. Along with the existing ORYX core measures, the library includes measures such as the intensive care unit and nursing-sensitive care measures. Over time, the measure reserve library will be expanded to include externally developed measures that have been evaluated by The Joint Commission against strict criteria. Each measure will include calculation algorithms and relevant data element definitions, and all sets will be submitted to the National Quality Forum for consideration and potential endorsement. More information and specifications are on the Joint Commission's Web site at http://www.jointcommission.org/library_of_other_measures.

Strategic Surveillance System

One of the most compelling needs of health care organizations is actionable data and information that can be used to prioritize and drive quality and safety improvement efforts. Toward that end, The Joint Commission developed the Strategic Surveillance System (S3), now provided as a value-added element of the accreditation process to help accredited hospitals identify and prioritize areas for improvement. (Although the eventual goal of S3 is to spread the concept to all of the Joint

Commission's accreditation programs, no date has been set to expand S3 beyond the hospital program.) S3 takes the data/information used in the Priority Focus Process and expands upon it, providing the hospital with the detail behind each priority focus area and clinical/service group identified as an area of risk and potential improvement. The S3 reports are provided through each hospital's password-protected *Joint Commission Connect* extranet site at no additional charge, but the data are not available to the public. The Priority Focus Area Dashboard Report provides a visual summary, highlighting areas for improvement that can be used in strategic planning processes and as a diagnostic tool to provide drill-down capability within the highlighted areas for improvement.

Hospitals can analyze comparative performance against national and state priority focus areas and clinical/service group data (as well as data from other specialized groups, such as magnet hospitals or hospitals that have received Contingent Accreditation or Preliminary Denial of Accreditation status). These information reports, continuously updated and provided to hospitals on a quarterly basis, are intended to serve as management tools that organizations can use to optimize system performance by focusing their energies and resources on identified vulnerable systems and services.

Overall, feedback from hospitals has shown that they appreciate the module's synthesis of large amounts of data into intelligent information, the comparative reporting and systems analysis, and the proactive identification of themes and trends. A user guide and a Web-based tutorial are also provided on *Joint Commission Connect*.

Patient Safety

The overall goal of accreditation and performance measurement is to reduce the risks to patients and ensure that they receive safe, high-quality care. The Joint Commission has built patient safety into all aspects of its accreditation process to help organizations incorporate it into all their improvement efforts.

Office of Quality Monitoring

The Joint Commission relies on information from a variety of sources—including patients and families, government agencies, the public, an organization's staff, and the media—to reinforce its oversight efforts and improve the quality and safety of care in accredited organizations. Such information often comes in the form of complaints. The Office of Quality Monitoring provides an easy way for anyone to contact The Joint Commission about standards-related quality-of-care issues in accredited organizations. Common complaints deal with issues such as rights, care, safety, staffing, and medication use.

The Joint Commission encourages anyone with safety or quality concerns or complaints to notify the health care organization's leaders first, which usually produces a more timely resolution of the matter. If the concern or complaint remains unresolved, it can be reported to the Office of Quality Monitoring by fax (630/792-5636), e-mail (complaint@jointcommission.org), online (http://jcwebnoc.jcaho.org/QMSInternet/IncidentEntry.aspx), or mail (Office of Quality Monitoring, The Joint Commission, One Renaissance Boulevard, Oakbrook Terrace, IL 60181). Because many people do not want to sign or give their names for fear of reprisals, the confidentiality of information provided by those calling or writing is strictly maintained. The office does not deal with billing, insurance, payment disputes, individual personnel, or labor relations issues. More information can be found at http://www.jointcommission.org/report_a_complaint.aspx.

Sentinel Event Policy

The Joint Commission's Sentinel Event Policy is designed to help organizations that experience serious adverse events in patient care to improve safety. The policy encourages voluntary reporting of sentinel events to The Joint Commission and requires that a root cause analysis be conducted for each of these "reviewable" events (*see* Sidebar 2-2 on page 55). Voluntary reporting of events has several advantages, including the following:

➤ Contributing to lessons learned that can be shared with other organizations experiencing similar events
➤ Sending a message to stakeholders that everything possible is being done to ensure that similar events are prevented
➤ Consulting with Joint Commission staff during root cause analysis and formation of an action plan

Sentinel events reported to The Joint Commission are included in its Sentinel Event Database. The Joint Commission publishes sentinel event statistics that can be accessed based on type of event, setting, reporting source, outcomes, self-report-

Chapter 2

> **Sidebar 2-2. Reviewable Sentinel Events**
>
> **Definition of a Sentinel Event:** An unexpected occurrence involving death or serious physical or psychological injury or risk thereof. (Serious injury specifically includes loss of limb or function.) The phrase "or risk thereof" includes any process variation for which a recurrence would carry a significant chance of a serious adverse outcome.
>
> **Reviewable Events:**
> - Suicide of any individual receiving care, treatment, or services in a staffed, around-the-clock care setting or within 72 hours of discharge
> - Unanticipated death of a full-term infant
> - Abduction of any individual receiving care, treatment, or services
> - Discharge of an infant to the wrong family
> - Rape
> - Hemolytic transfusion reaction involving the administration of blood or blood products having major blood group incompatibilities (ABO, Rh, and other blood groups)
> - Surgical and nonsurgical invasive procedure on the wrong patient or wrong site, or wrong procedure*
> - Unintended retention of a foreign object in an individual after surgery or another procedure
> - Severe neonatal hyperbilirubinemia (bilirubin > 30 milligrams/deciliter)
> - Prolonged fluoroscopy with a cumulative dose > 1,500 rads to a single field or any delivery of radiotherapy to the wrong body region or at > 25% above the planned radiotherapy dose
>
> * All events of surgery on the wrong patient or wrong body part are reviewable under the policy, regardless of the magnitude of the procedure or the outcome.

ed events by year, and method for review of organization response. The information from this database can be used to study the underlying causes of events, share experiences with other health care organizations, and reduce the risk of future adverse events.

To raise the awareness of both the health care field and the federal government about sentinel events and how they can be prevented, The Joint Commission periodically publishes *Sentinel Event Alert*s, which are accessible at http://www.jointcommission.org/sentinel_event.aspx. The issues covered in the newsletter are prompted by results from the database of reported incidents, and the recommendations for reducing risks are developed from the experiences of actual organizations and from the advice of experts in the field. Recent topics have included preventing inpatient suicide, violence in the health care setting, and maternal deaths.

National Patient Safety Goals

The Joint Commission developed its first set of National Patient Safety Goals in 2002. The goals were based on data obtained from the Joint Commission's Sentinel Event Database and were recommended by a panel of patient safety experts. Although the first National Patient Safety Goals were applicable only to hospitals, goals have since been developed for each accreditation program. Each goal is accompanied by elements of performance (much like standards), and compliance with the elements of performance is required for accreditation.

In 2003 The Joint Commission created the Universal Protocol for Preventing Wrong Site, Wrong Procedure, Wrong Person Surgery™ to address the persistence of these types of medical errors. Applicable to all operative and other invasive procedures performed in accredited hospitals, critical access hospitals, ambulatory care organizations, and office-based surgery practices, the Universal Protocol has three main components:

1. A preoperative verification that all relevant documentation and studies are available; have been reviewed; and are consistent with each other, the patient's expectations, and the surgical team's understanding of the procedure to be performed
2. Marking of the operative site to ensure unambiguous identification of the intended site of incision or insertion
3. A "time-out" immediately before starting the procedure, during which all members of the surgical/procedure team resolve any questions or concerns and do a final verification of the correct patient, procedure, and site

The protocol has been endorsed by nearly 30 professional health care associations and organizations. (*See* the elements of performance for the Universal Protocol and National Patient Safety Goals for 2011 in Sidebar 2-3 on page 57.)

Sidebar 2-3. Hospital National Patient Safety Goals for 2011[1]

Goal 1: Improve the accuracy of patient identification.
NPSG.01.01.01: Use at least two patient identifiers when providing care, treatment, and services.
NPSG.01.03.01: Eliminate transfusion errors related to patient misidentification.

Goal 2: Improve the effectiveness of communication among caregivers.
NPSG.02.03.01: Report critical results of tests and diagnostic procedures on a timely basis.

Goal 3: Improve the safety of using medications.
NPSG.03.04.01: Label all medications, medication containers, and other solutions on and off the sterile field in perioperative and other procedural settings.
NPSG.03.05.01: Reduce the likelihood of patient harm associated with the use of anticoagulation therapy.
NPSG.03.06.01: Maintain and communicate accurate medication information.*

Goal 7: Reduce the risk of health care–associated infections.
NPSG.07.01.01: Comply with either current Centers for Disease Control and Prevention (CDC) hand hygiene guidelines or World Health Organization (WHO) hand hygiene guidelines.
NPSG.07.03.01: Implement evidence-based practices to prevent health care–associated infections due to multidrug-resistant organisms in acute care hospitals.
NPSG.07.04.01: Implement best practices or evidence-based guidelines to prevent central line–associated bloodstream infections.
NPSG.07.05.01: Implement best practices for prevention of surgical site infections.

Goal 15: The organization identifies safety risks inherent in its patient population.
NPSG.15.01.01: Identify patients at risk for suicide.

Universal Protocol: The organization fulfills the expectations set forth in the Universal Protocol.
UP.01.01.01: Conduct a preprocedure verification process.
UP.01.02.01: Mark the procedure site.
UP.01.03.01: A time-out is performed before the procedure.

---

* The revised medication reconciliation requirements under NPSG.03.06.01 (previously National Patient Safety Goal 8) become effective July 1, 2011.

The Joint Commission Center for Transforming Healthcare

The Joint Commission Center for Transforming Healthcare was established in 2009 with the goal of solving health care's most critical safety and quality problems. The Center develops solutions, in partnership with the nation's leading health care systems, using Robust Process Improvement™ (RPI), which incorporates tools and methods such as Lean Six Sigma. Through the Center, leading health care organizations have joined together in project teams to address the following critical issues, with more to come in the future:

- Hand hygiene
- Hand-off communications
- Correct site, procedure, and person surgery
- Surgical site infections

In 2010 The Joint Commission launched the Targeted Solutions Tool™, which implements the work of the participating organizations and the Joint Commission Center for Transforming Healthcare by providing a step-by-step guide to the following actions:

- Measure performance.
- Identify barriers to the expected performance.
- Implement proven solutions.

The first set of targeted solutions, created by eight of the country's leading health care organizations along with the Center for Transforming Healthcare, focused on improving hand hygiene. The Center is also developing targeted solutions for hand-off communication, wrong-site surgery, and surgical site infections.

For more information about the Center for Transforming Healthcare, go to http://www.centerfortransforminghealthcare.org.

Patient Education

Although there has been a push in recent years to involve patients more fully in their own treatment and care, they are sometimes overlooked as integral members of the health care team in preventing errors. In 2002 The Joint Commission and

CMS introduced a national program called Speak Up™, which encourages patient participation in improving safety. Health care organizations can purchase materials such as posters, buttons, and brochures to distribute to patients at http://www.jcrinc.com/other-resources, or select materials can be downloaded free of charge from http://www.jointcommission.org/speakup.aspx. Patients should be given easy-to-understand information about specific safety issues, suggestions for ways they can reduce risks, and potential questions to ask their health care team. In addition to the initial offering, titled *Speak Up: Help Prevent Errors in Your Care,* materials for these topics are also available:

- *Tips for Your Doctor's Visit*
- *Understanding Your Doctors and Other Caregivers*
- *Know Your Rights*
- *Reduce Your Risk of Falling*
- *Prevent Errors in Your Child's Care*
- *What You Should Know About Pain Management*
- *What You Should Know About Research Studies*
- *Help Avoid Mistakes in Your Surgery*
- *Information for Living Organ Donors*
- *Five Things You Can Do to Prevent Infection*
- *Help Prevent Medical Test Mistakes*
- *Help Avoid Mistakes with Your Medicines*
- *Planning Your Follow-Up Care*
- *Diabetes: Five Ways to Be Active in Your Care at the Hospital*
- *Dialysis: Five Ways to Be Active in Your Care at the Hospital*
- *Help Prevent Errors in Your Care*
- *Stay Well and Keep Others Well* (a Speak Up coloring book for kids)

Published in 2006, *YOU: The Smart Patient: An Insider's Handbook for Getting the Best Treatment** educates readers about how to take control of their own health care

---

* Roizen M.F., Oz M.C., Joint Commission: *YOU: The Smart Patient: An Insider's Handbook for Getting the Best Treatment.* New York: The Free Press, 2006.

and that of their families. This book helps patients deal with issues such as choosing the right physician, hospital, and insurance company and helps them make decisions regarding prescription drugs, specialists, treatment options, alternative medicine, and pain management. Using humor and illustrations, this book provides patients with concrete guidance in finding their way through the health care system and urges them to become involved in their own care. Readers learn about how the National Patient Safety Goals, Quality Check, and the Universal Protocol can help them evaluate health care organizations; how to use the "Patient's Health Journal"; and what to do when they require care in a foreign country.

Published in 2010, *The Smart Parent's Guide to Getting Your Kids Through Checkups, Illnesses, and Accidents* is the Joint Commission's and Joint Commission Resources' second book produced specifically for the public. The Joint Commission and Joint Commission Resources collaborated on this book with Jennifer Trachtenberg, M.D., a nationally renowned parenting expert and board-certified pediatrician. The book is available online from a variety of vendors.

Quality Check®

Transparency in reporting on the performance of health care organizations is vital to giving consumers and employers the information they need to make informed decisions, to maintaining the trust of the public, and to motivating organizations to continuously push for better safety and quality. The Joint Commission provides organization-specific performance information to the public via its Quality Check Web site (http://www.qualitycheck.org). Quality Check allows users to search for organizations by name, geographic location, or type of services (such as acute care) and provides information on the following:

- Accreditation status
- Standards compliance problem areas
- Distinctive organization achievements (special quality awards or merit badges)
- Comparative performance data for National Quality Improvement Goals (core measures), National Patient Safety Goals, patient mortality, and hospital readmission rates

Much of the information available through Quality Check is also shown on an organization's Quality Report (*see* Figure 2-1, pages 61–69), which is available after

Chapter 2

its triennial survey and details both the facility's performance and how it compares to that of similar organizations. Such comparisons can help leaders identify where they may need to concentrate improvement efforts. This report is also evidence of Joint Commission accreditation, which can be used as a strong marketing tool to demonstrate the organization's commitment to and advances in safety and quality to patients, insurers, and others.

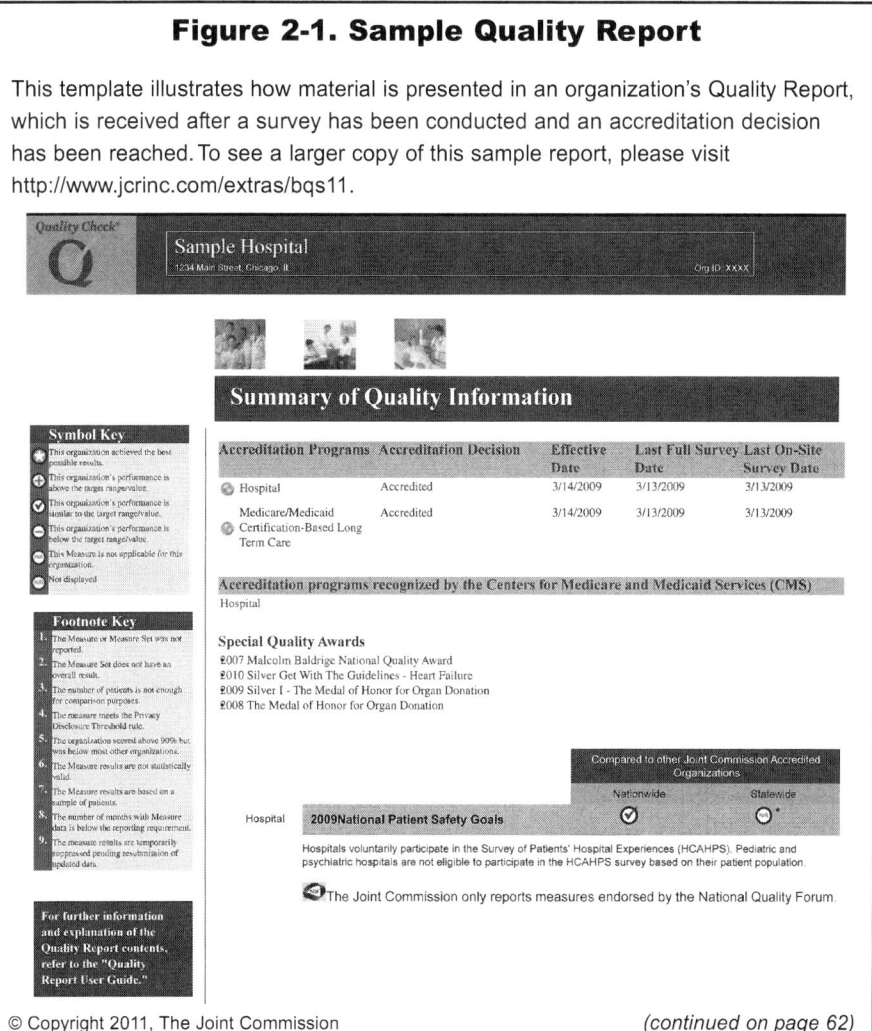

Figure 2-1. Sample Quality Report

This template illustrates how material is presented in an organization's Quality Report, which is received after a survey has been conducted and an accreditation decision has been reached. To see a larger copy of this sample report, please visit http://www.jcrinc.com/extras/bqs11.

© Copyright 2011, The Joint Commission

(continued on page 62)

Getting the Board on Board

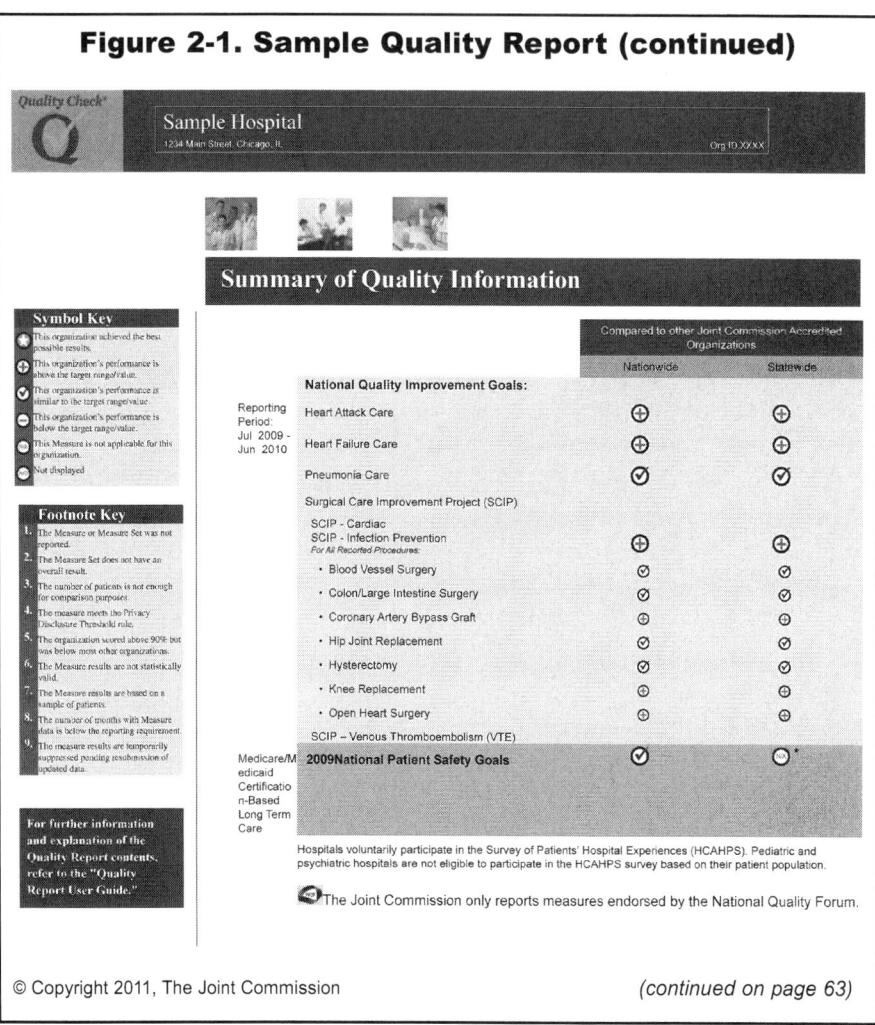

Figure 2-1. Sample Quality Report (continued)

(continued on page 63)

Chapter 2

Figure 2-1. Sample Quality Report (continued)

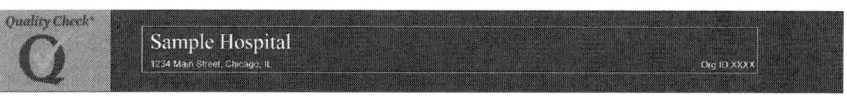

Sample Hospital
1234 Main Street, Chicago, IL
Org ID XXXX

Locations of Care

* Primary Location

Locations of Care	Available Services	
Sample Hospital **1234 Main Street** **Chicago, IL 60614**	• Cancer Center/Oncology (Inpatient, Outpatient) • Cardiac Catheterization Lab (Inpatient) • Cardiac Surgery (Inpatient) • Cardiac Unit/Cardiology (Inpatient, Outpatient) • CT Scanner (Inpatient, Outpatient) • Dialysis (Inpatient) • EEG/EKG/EMG Lab (Inpatient, Outpatient) • Emergency Room (Outpatient) • Gastroenterology (Inpatient, Outpatient) • General Medical Services (Inpatient) • General Surgery (Inpatient, Outpatient) • GI or Endoscopy Lab (Inpatient, Outpatient) • Gynecology (Inpatient, Outpatient) • Imaging/Radiology (Inpatient, Outpatient) • Infectious Diseases (Inpatient) • Infusion Therapy (Inpatient, Outpatient) • Intensive Care Unit (Inpatient) • Labor & Delivery (Inpatient) • Lithotripsy/Kidney Stone Treatment (Inpatient, Outpatient) • Long Term Care • Magnetic Resonance Imaging (Inpatient, Outpatient) • Neonatal Intensive Care (Inpatient) • Nephrology (Inpatient) • Neurology (Inpatient) • Neurosurgery (Inpatient) • Nuclear Medicine (Inpatient, Outpatient)	• Nursery (Inpatient) • Obstetrics (Inpatient) • Operating Room (Inpatient, Outpatient) • Ophthalmology/Eye Surgery (Inpatient) • Oral Maxillofacial Surgery (Inpatient) • Orthopedic Surgery (Inpatient, Outpatient) • Otolaryngology/Ear, Nose, and Throat (Inpatient, Outpatient) • Outpatient Surgery (Outpatient) • Pain Management (Outpatient) • Plastic Surgery (Inpatient, Outpatient) • Post Anesthesia Care Unit (PACU) (Inpatient, Outpatient) • Pulmonary Function Lab (Inpatient, Outpatient) • Radiation Oncology (Inpatient, Outpatient) • Recovery/Infirmary (Outpatient) • Rehabilitation and Physical Medicine (Inpatient, Outpatient) • Rehabilitation Services • Respiratory Care (Ventilator) (Inpatient) • Skilled Nursing Care • Skilled Nursing Facility (Inpatient) • Telemetry (Inpatient) • Thoracic Surgery (Inpatient) • Ultrasound (Inpatient, Outpatient) • Urgent Care/Emergency Medicine (Outpatient) • Vascular Surgery (Inpatient) • Wound Care (Inpatient)
Sample Outpatient **Services** **4321 Main Street** **Chicago, IL 60641**	• Ambulatory Surgery Center (Outpatient) • Anesthesia (Outpatient)	

© Copyright 2011, The Joint Commission

(continued on page 64)

Getting the Board on Board

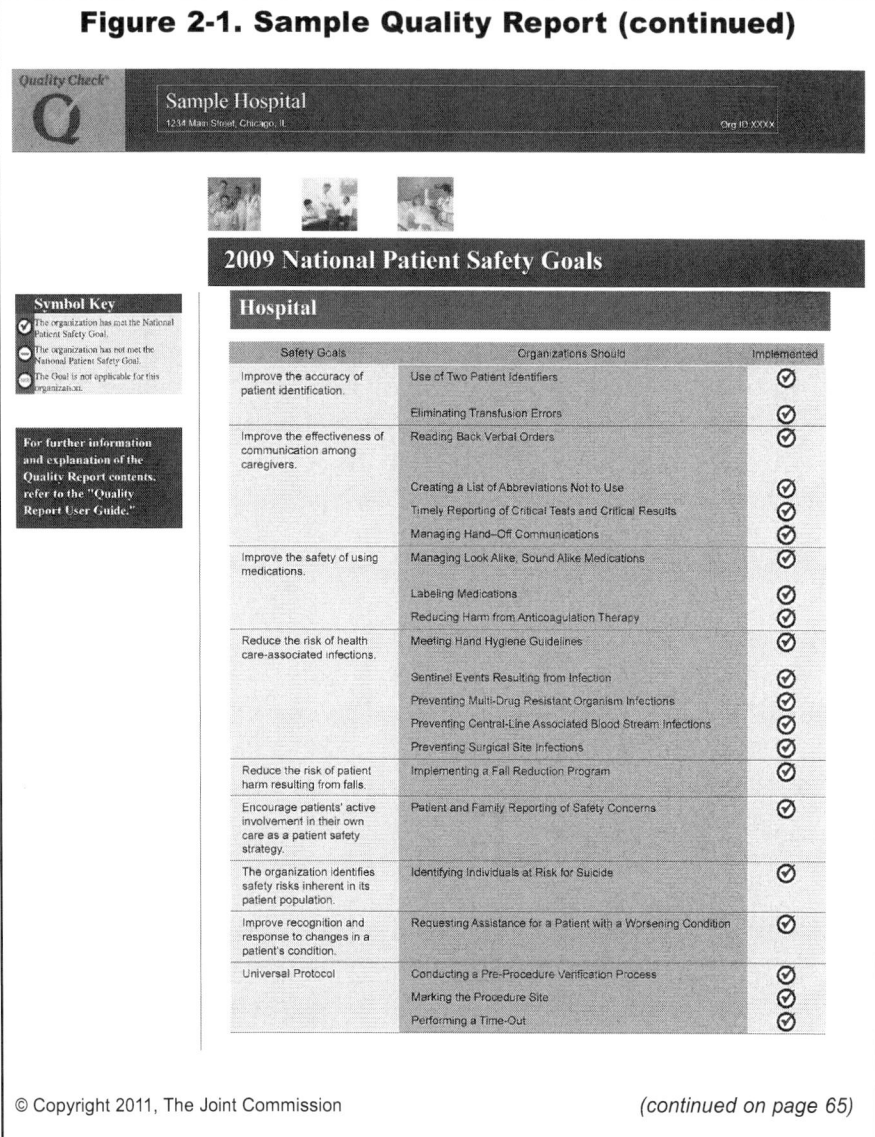

Figure 2-1. Sample Quality Report (continued)

(continued on page 65)

Chapter 2

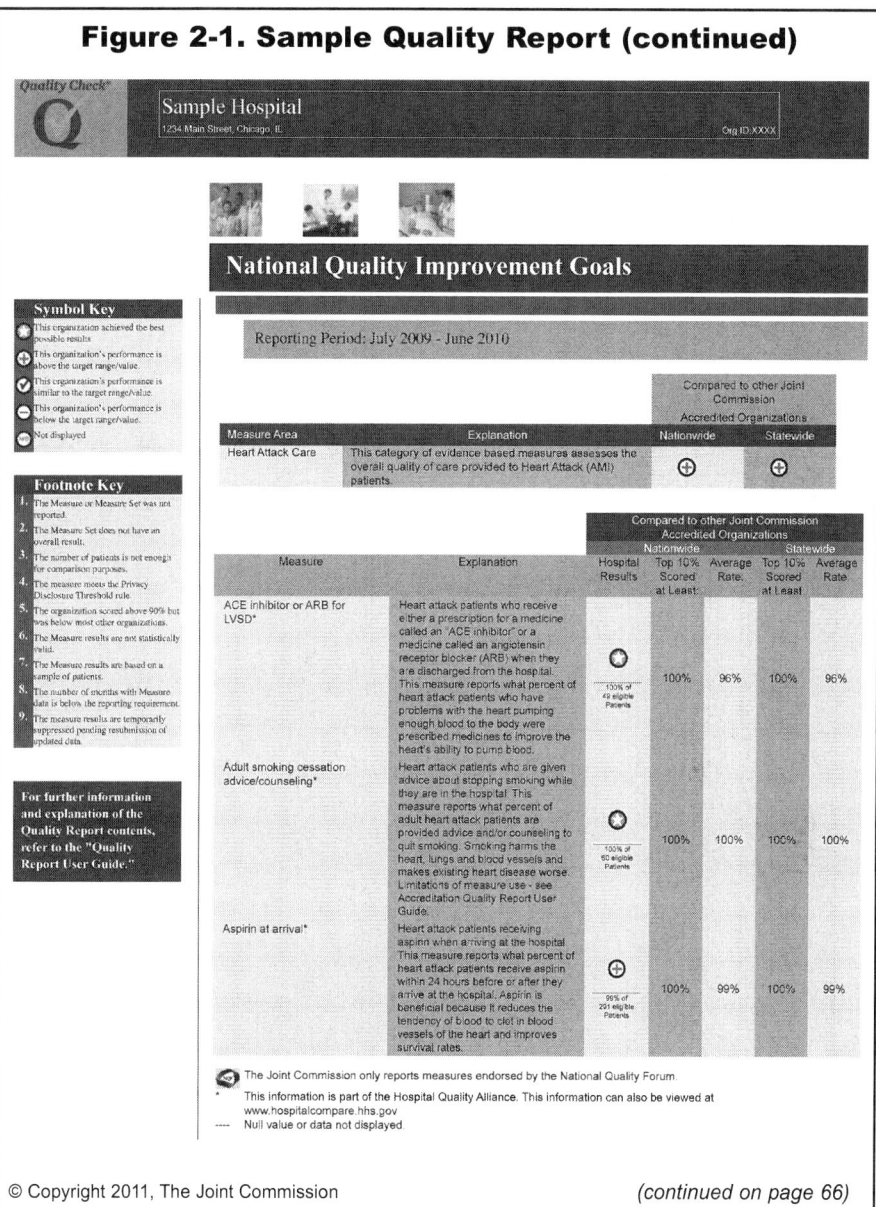

Figure 2-1. Sample Quality Report (continued)

(continued on page 66)

Getting the Board on Board

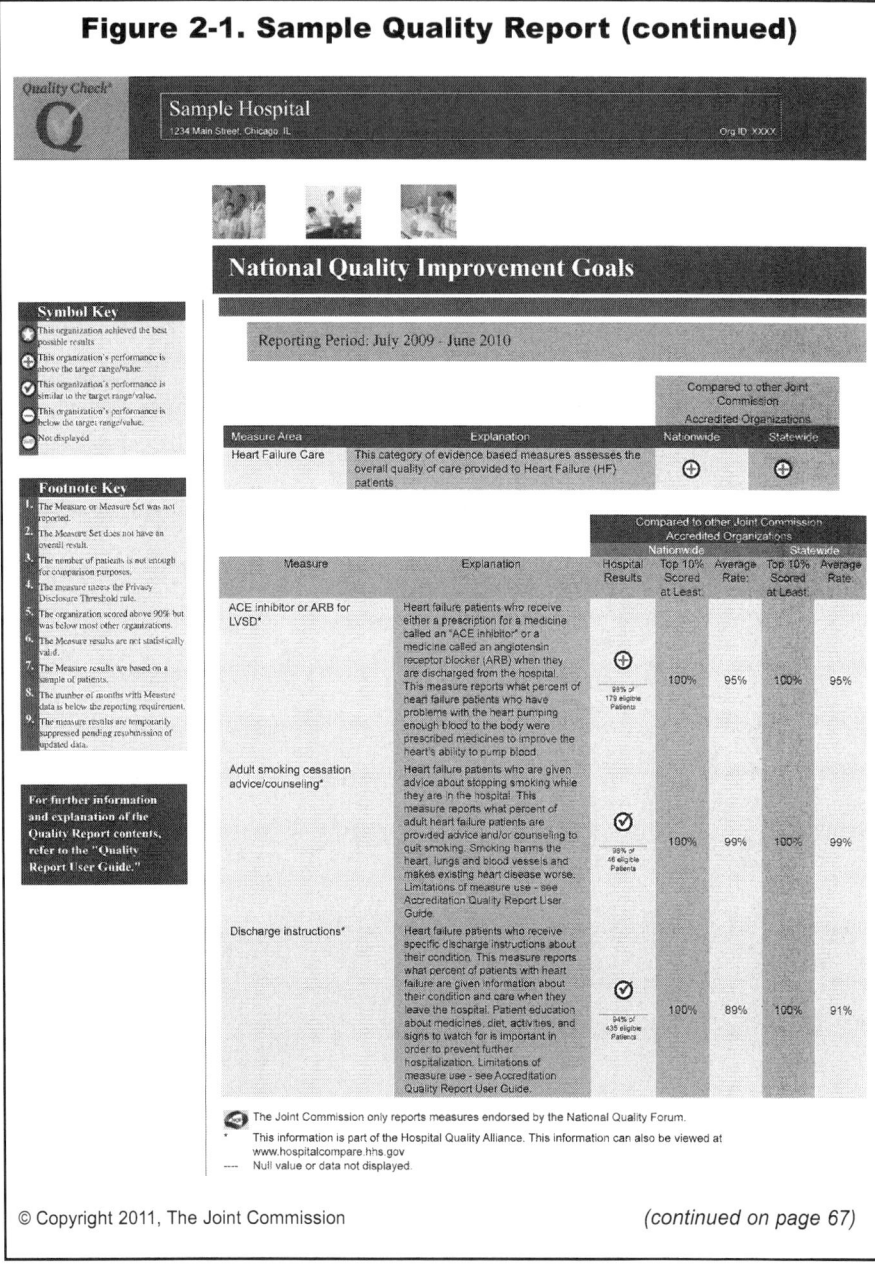

Figure 2-1. Sample Quality Report (continued)

(continued on page 67)

Chapter 2

Figure 2-1. Sample Quality Report (continued)

Quality Check®

Sample Hospital
1234 Main Street, Chicago, IL
Org ID: XXXX

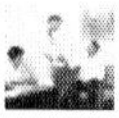

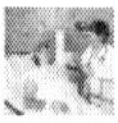

CMS Mortality Rates

Hospital

For further information and explanation of the Quality Report contents, refer to the "Quality Report User Guide."

Center for Medicare and Medicaid (CMS) Hospital 30-Day Risk Adjusted Death (Mortality) compared to U.S. National Rate
The rates displayed in this table are from data reported for discharges July 2006 through June 2009
Last Updated: October 07, 2010

The U.S. National 30-day Death Rate from Heart Attack = 16%			
	Better Than U.S. National Rate (Adjusted mortality is lower than U.S. rate)	No Different Than U.S. National Rate (Adjusted mortality is about the same as U.S. rate or difference is uncertain)	Worse Than U.S. National Rate (Adjusted mortality is higher than U.S. Rate)
30-Day Death (Mortality) Rates from Heart Attack = **18.3%**	Not Available		
Number of Medicare Heart Attack Patients = 237			
Out of 4569 hospitals in U.S.	95 hospitals in the U.S. Better than U.S. National Rate	2744 hospitals in the U.S. No different than U.S. National Rate	45 hospitals in the U.S. Worse than U.S. National Rate
	1685 hospitals in the United States did not have enough cases to reliably tell how well they are performing		
Out of 333 hospitals in state	4 hospitals in state Better than U.S. National Rate	228 hospitals in state No different than U.S. National Rate	2 hospitals in state Worse than U.S. National Rate
	99 hospitals in state did not have enough cases to reliably tell how well they are performing		

The U.S. National 30-day Death Rate from Heart Failure = 11%			
	Better Than U.S. National Rate (Adjusted mortality is lower than U.S. rate)	No Different Than U.S. National Rate (Adjusted mortality is about the same as U.S. rate or difference is uncertain)	Worse Than U.S. National Rate (Adjusted mortality is higher than U.S. Rate)
30-Day Death (Mortality) Rates from Heart Failure = **8.5%**	Not Available		
Number of Medicare Heart Failure Patients = 467			
Out of 4743 hospitals in U.S.	199 hospitals in the U.S. Better than U.S. National Rate	3801 hospitals in the U.S. No different than U.S. National Rate	140 hospitals in the U.S. Worse than U.S. National Rate
	603 hospitals in the United States did not have enough cases to reliably tell how well they are performing		
Out of 346 hospitals in state	13 hospitals in state Better than U.S. National Rate	267 hospitals in state No different than U.S. National Rate	11 hospitals in state Worse than U.S. National Rate
	55 hospitals in state did not have enough cases to reliably tell how well they are performing		

The U.S. National 30-day Death Rate from Pneumonia = 12%			
	Better Than U.S. National Rate (Adjusted mortality is lower than U.S. rate)	No Different Than U.S. National Rate (Adjusted mortality is about the same as U.S. rate or difference is uncertain)	Worse Than U.S. National Rate (Adjusted mortality is higher than U.S. Rate)
30-Day Death (Mortality) Rates from Pneumonia = **10.6%**	Not Available		
Number of Medicare Pneumonia Patients = 369			

© Copyright 2011, The Joint Commission   *(continued on page 68)*

Getting the Board on Board

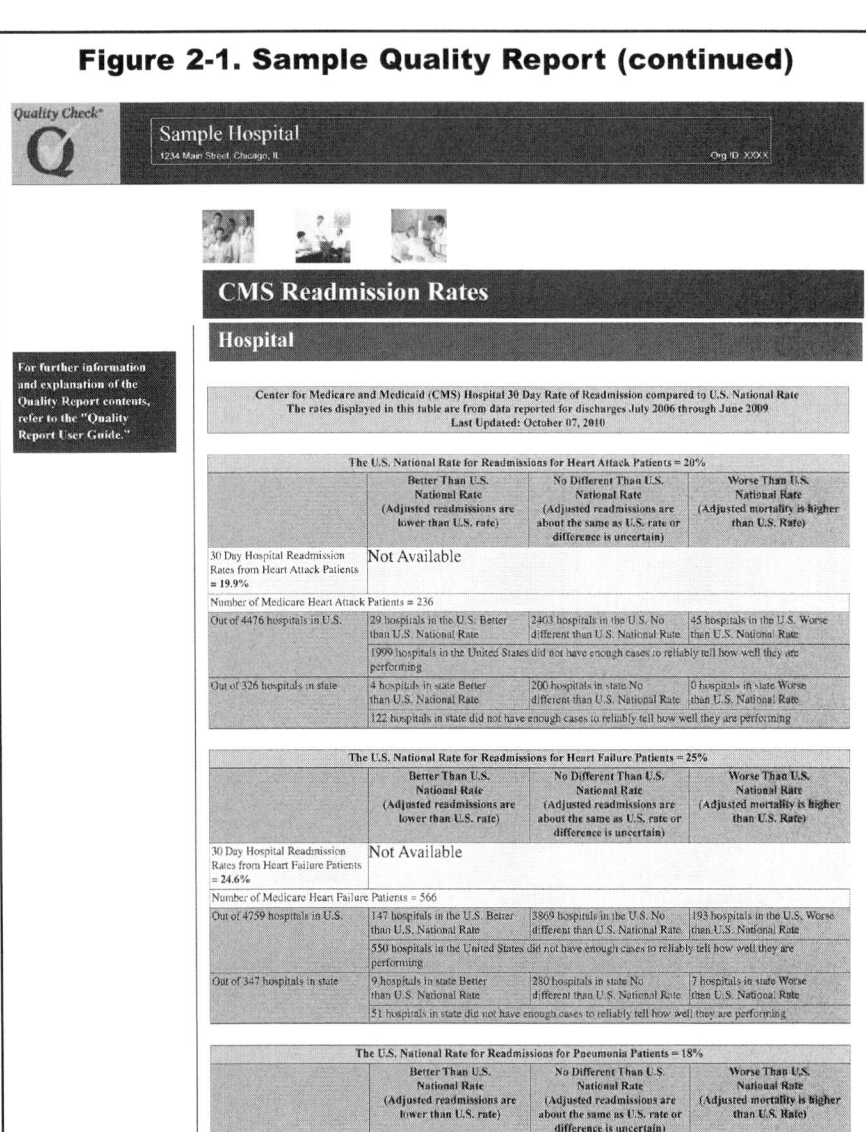

Chapter 2

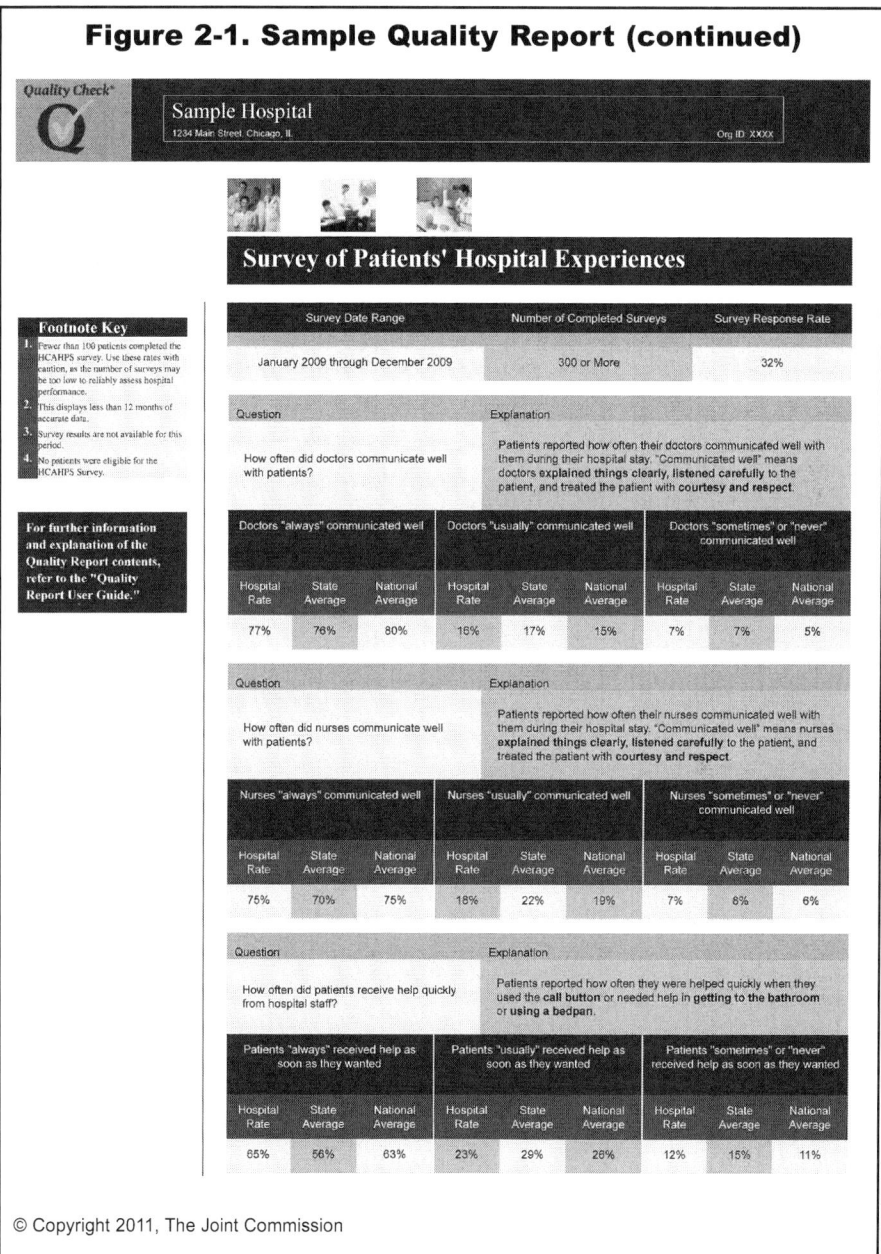

Figure 2-1. Sample Quality Report (continued)

© Copyright 2011, The Joint Commission

69

The Next Step

Armed with knowledge of national safety and quality efforts and an understanding of how The Joint Commission works with health care organizations to improve the safety and quality of care, you are now ready to take on the challenge of addressing these issues in your own facility or system. Chapter 3 offers suggestions and examples from actual health care organizations in which board members effectively discharge their leadership responsibilities and help create a culture of safety and quality.

Reference

1. The Joint Commission: *2011 Comprehensive Accreditation Manual for Hospitals: The Official Handbook.* Oak Brook, IL: Joint Commission Resources, 2010.

Chapter 3
The Board's Role in Improving Quality and Safety

Whether you are a new or long-standing board member, you may feel uncomfortable dealing with topics that have traditionally been categorized as clinical, medical, or administrative concerns. Board members without medical or health care backgrounds may be especially reluctant to give opinions. "Board members tend to be afraid of addressing quality and safety issues because they think, 'I'm a layperson. What do I know about quality and safety?'" notes Lee Carter, long-time trustee at Cincinnati Children's Hospital Medical Center in Ohio. "While the board is not going to reduce surgical site infections or codes outside the intensive care unit themselves, they can shine a light on problems and ask people, 'What is the benchmark? What is the target? How are we doing in reaching the target?' By asking those questions, they focus the staff's and administration's attention in a way that may not happen if the board is not involved." To help address problems in care, board members across hospitals can share the safety improvement mechanisms their own organizations use for identifying and reducing exposure to risks.

In the ever-changing world of health care, the role of the board member may seem difficult to define. Escalating costs, regulatory demands for transparency and accountability, public demands for better and safer care, and corporate demands for better profits all jockey for priority. As a member of your institution's board, you need to understand the board's fiduciary, medical, and legal responsibilities and how you can best meet them. "You're basically attesting that the quality of care in your organization is at the level it should be; that medical staff are discharging their responsibilities to engage in appropriate peer review and credentialing; and that management has provided for a safe and protective environment for its patients, staff, and family members," explains Jeffrey Brickman, F.A.C.H.E., system senior vice president and president and CEO for Provena Saint Joseph Medical Center, Joliet, Illinois. "Once board members understand that, it opens the door for them to ask, 'What does that mean for me?'"

Many boards establish a separate committee or group dedicated to reviewing only quality and safety issues; this committee then reports back to the full board on sentinel events, measurement and improvement activities, and so on. The quality committee may include trustees, senior hospital leaders, department directors, and/or patient and family representatives. The key point is that this group of individuals focuses on the organization's approach to quality and safety, the integration of this approach throughout all areas, and the process used to improve care at the organization. For example, the CEO and the board chair of Sentara Healthcare, a system that serves southeastern Virginia and northeastern North Carolina, strongly believe that anyone who is going to head the board of directors should have a thorough understanding of quality, safety, and medical staff affairs. To this end, they have instituted a policy that requires each board chair to first serve as the chairperson of the board's quality subcommittee.

A recent survey of 722 chairpersons found that 63% of hospital boards discuss quality improvement issues at each meeting, and this discussion comprises at least 20% of the agenda for more than half the boards.[1] Furthermore, three out of five boards have a quality subcommittee, and 72% regularly review a quality dashboard. Finally, more than half of hospital board members rated quality of care as a top priority.[1] Regardless of whether your board already makes quality and safety issues a high priority or still focuses primarily on financial responsibilities, there are ways to become more involved and make a difference in your organization:

- ▶ Promote a culture of quality and safety.
- ▶ Participate in measurement and improvement.
- ▶ Hold management accountable for change.
- ▶ Address quality and safety issues in board meetings.

A study by the Agency for Healthcare Research and Quality found that when governing boards are involved in quality and safety, their organizations' mortality rates decrease and they see better performance in processes of care.[2] Moreover, the following board functions were associated with better outcomes across the organization[2]:

- Establishing a board quality committee
- Setting strategic goals for quality improvement
- Participating in setting the quality agenda for the hospital
- Discussing a specific goal for quality in board meetings
- Tracking the organization's performance with dashboards that include national benchmarks for clinical quality, patient safety, and patient satisfaction
- Tying senior executives' performance evaluation to quality and patient safety indicators

As your board gives more attention to quality and safety, the rest of your organization will follow suit.

Promoting a Culture of Quality and Safety

An organizational culture that focuses on learning and takes a proactive approach to improving safety and quality is a goal of many systems and facilities. Because of the complexities of cultural change, patience, dedication, and top-down support are required. Staff may be resistant to reporting errors, taking part in measurement and improvement activities, and/or establishing and learning new processes. Leaders may want greater transparency and improved quality but may be uncomfortable with problems that are uncovered through reporting and measurement. The temptation to maintain the status quo is high—but this is where board members can push for change, setting the tone for a culture that does not tolerate patients' exposure to harm.

Transparency and honest communication are the keys to developing a proactive culture of quality and safety. By recognizing that improvement efforts will expose defects within your processes that are actually opportunities for improvement, you can encourage the administration to look for defects rather than avoid them. Let your organization's leaders know that you expect them to identify and address problems without worrying about "how things look." Make it known that your priority is delivering safe, high-quality care to patients, and encourage managers and staff to be candid about what is actually happening (or not happening) within the organization.

Leaders across your organization will take their cues from you when it comes to making quality and safety a part of daily operations. You should promote organizationwide education and training for staff and leaders so that everyone understands the principles of quality and the measures necessary for preventing safety risks to patients and staff alike. "When your board chair and board members are behind change, it helps move things along," says Richard Davis, Ph.D., executive director of Johns Hopkins Medicine Center for Innovation in Quality Patient Care in Baltimore. "For example, our board chair understands that over the last few years, we've been pushing the need to incorporate quality and safety into every element of hospital operations across our health system. He and the board require regular and detailed updates on our progress with this initiative. This kind of focus can give administration the leverage we sometimes need to remove some of the barriers that may have been challenging in the past."

Education is also important for board members. A recent survey found that only 32% of hospital boards had received any formal training in clinical quality.[1] If you feel that you or other members of your board do not have the requisite knowledge to participate fully in discussions about quality and safety, ask administration for more information and training. Many organizations urge trustees to attend conferences and lectures on quality and safety; others arrange retreats where board members can talk with quality experts in health care and other fields, explore national and organizational trends, and look at key trouble spots within the organization in more depth than is possible at monthly or quarterly meetings. To keep its board highly educated, Banner Health, headquartered in Phoenix, invites experts in the patient safety and quality improvement field to speak with the board and sends packets of safety and quality articles between board meetings. (For more information on how Banner Health's board gets involved in patient safety and quality improvement, *see* the case study on pages 75–77.)

Even if your board is already familiar with quality and safety, continuing education can often suggest new areas for consideration or raise the level of expectations for improvement. For example, the board members of Iowa Health System, which operates facilities throughout the state, were already familiar with quality and safety initiatives when Donald Berwick, M.D., M.P.P.H., then president and CEO of the Institute for Healthcare Improvement, came to talk to them. That discussion accelerated the board's interest in quality. A board retreat was held approximately six

Chapter 3

months later, and the stories told and advice given by experts there gave the board members a pattern for the kind of quality work they wanted to see implemented in their system. It prompted them to request a multiyear proposal for a systemwide set of initiatives that would take some of the high-level clinical processes present in all system hospitals and raise the common performance level.

CASE STUDY: BANNER HEALTH

Banner Health, a nonprofit hospital system based in Phoenix, is made up of 23 hospitals and health care facilities across seven states (Alaska, Arizona, California, Colorado, Nebraska, Nevada, and Wyoming). The 15 members of Banner Health's board meet quarterly for two days and are ultimately accountable for quality and safety. In 2001 Banner Health's board developed and adopted its mission statement, which is to "make a difference in people's lives through excellent patient care." As John Hensing, M.D., executive vice president and chief medical officer, reports, "Whenever they are making decisions, the board reminds itself of this important mission." Ten of the board members sit on the Board Care Management and Quality Committee. "The board members on the quality committee review Banner Health's strategic initiatives and global performance from a quality perspective," says Hensing.

Every year Banner Health approves a set of strategic initiatives, 30%–40% of which typically involve clinical/patient safety goals. "In 2006 Banner Health set strategic initiatives that involved reaching upper quartile performance in clinical quality metrics, such as heart failure, acute myocardial infarction, surgical care, and pneumonia," says Hensing. "We've progressively worked our way toward achieving that initiative and are currently in the 80th percentile in all those metrics. We've also been recognized by Thomson Reuters as one of the top 10 health systems in the country for clinical quality and performance in the core measures." In addition to these goals for clinical outcomes, Banner Health has identified goals for patient safety, including a reduction in the following:

- Central line infections
- Hospital-acquired conditions

- Uterine tachysystole due to oxytocin
- Reoperative bleeds after coronary artery bypass graft surgeries

Allocating Resources for Quality

To achieve its strategic initiatives, Banner Health must have sufficient resources. "As chief medical officer, I enjoy a very supportive and engaged board that has made major resource and allocation decisions for investments to improve Banner's quality and patient safety," says Hensing. Recent investments that the board has approved in order to improve patient safety include the following:

- A 55,000-square-foot simulation medical center in Mesa, Arizona
- An electronic intensive care unit system
- An electronic medical record system
- An obstetrical clinical decision support system

Educating Board Members

Banner Health's board members come from a variety of backgrounds, including medical, financial, laboratory, and information technology. Although each board member brings individual expertise to Banner Health, some may have limited knowledge of clinical and quality improvement issues. "We want to keep our board highly educated," says Hensing, "so we provide them with various resources for information regarding health care issues in general, clinical quality, and patient safety."

When a new board member is oriented to his or her role, patient safety and clinical quality are discussed at length. Thereafter, Banner Health provides ongoing education through presentations during board meetings from internal leaders or external speakers with expertise in patient safety and quality. "For example, we recently had speakers come to the board meeting to discuss the concepts of a 'just culture,'" says Hensing. In addition, leaders at Banner Health mail board members packets of articles between board meetings to keep them informed about new issues in health care and patient safety.

Holding Executives Accountable

Because the board is ultimately accountable for quality and patient safety, it must ensure that Banner Health meets its strategic initiatives. "The management of Banner Health is rewarded for achieving these strategic initiatives," says Hensing. "Of all the strategic initiatives, 40% are related to clinical or patient safety issues. We benchmark ourselves against national performance [such as the Total Benchmark Solution CMS Quality Management], and the goal is to achieve upper quartile performance. Overall, our success depends on meeting those strategic initiatives."

Engaging in Patient-Centered Activities

Often one of the most important ways you can affect organizational culture is to take part in activities that bring you into contact with patients and staff. One example is Patient Safety Leadership WalkRounds™, first instituted at Brigham and Women's Hospital in Boston, during which senior leaders and clinical leaders visit various areas of the organization and talk to staff members. These conversations may take place in hallways or more private areas, and they cover only safety issues. The leader explains to staff that the organization is focused on system problems and that no reprisals or blame will be directed toward those who report errors and close calls. He or she then asks open-ended questions about safety-related events or concerns and listens to the staff response. By limiting the discussion topic, the leader demonstrates his or her commitment to safety and helps to promote a nonpunitive culture.[3] This example from Brigham and Women's Hospital suggests that participating in walkarounds helps executives witness the effects of budgetary decisions on actual operations—that is, it helps them see how decisions made at the administrative end could lead to events of patient harm. Seeing the direct effect of actions, as opposed to discussing them in the abstract, can constitute a powerful inducement to change.[3]

Walkarounds—or any other activities that get leaders involved with patients and staff—need to be supported by a set of steps to document discussions, identify contributing factors related to each comment, and designate subsequent actions, such as reports provided to senior leadership and the board.[4] Yet board members themselves may find it beneficial to occasionally participate in the walkarounds. Not only do you learn firsthand what happens on the front lines of patient care, where providers experience problems with processes, and how patients and families feel about the care they receive, but you can also ask questions and bring up issues that may give managers and staff a new perspective. Similarly, shadowing a physician or another health care professional can be an eye-opening experience for trustees. According to Vincent O'Reilly, vice chair on the board for the Dana-Farber Cancer Institute in Boston, "You need a patient-centric organization and culture. Going on rounds makes it all real. For those of us who have done it, it has given us a lasting connection to the institute. We're dealing with cancer patients, and when I participated with two other trustees, we went on pediatric rounds. It was 25 or 30 years ago, but we still talk about it. It puts everything in perspective." (For more information on how Dana-Farber's board of directors is involved in quality and patient safety, *see* the case study on pages 80–85.)

After, or instead of, participating in walkarounds, you might want to sponsor or be involved in a specific safety or quality initiative. Depending on your background, you may be particularly interested in improving medication safety, preventing health care–associated infections in the intensive care unit, or meeting federal requirements for Medicare reimbursement. At The Johns Hopkins Hospital, the chairman of the quality committee of the board of trustees adopted a unit in the executive rounding program, and he participates in the unit's improvement projects. Because the chairman doesn't live in Maryland, administration partnered him with an on-site executive who can meet with unit staff on short notice or in the months when the board member is not in town. He participates by phone as needed. "This board member is exposed to some of the raw issues facing the people on the front line," says Lori Paine, R.N., M.S., director, patient safety. "We've been looking at delays in peaks and troughs of antibiotic therapy on that particular unit, tracking how communication happens between house staff and unit staff when they change services on a monthly basis, problems with storage, and noise on the unit." Having a board member who remains interested and involved in improvement efforts lets both staff and leaders know that such efforts are a high priority within the organization.

There are many other ways of showing your support for a culture of quality and safety. You might ask staff members working in an area that needs improvement to speak at a quality committee or board meeting to get a better idea of what the

Chapter 3

✪ Trustees Taking the Lead ✪

In 2004 the Centers for Medicare & Medicaid Services (CMS) and Premier, Inc., began a demonstration project called the Premier Hospital Quality Incentive Demonstration. Hospitals and systems were invited to submit quality data on more than 30 quality measures related to five clinical conditions, and the results were publicly reported on the CMS Web site. Hospitals whose performance was in the top 10th (decile) for a given set of measures received a 2% bonus payment in addition to standard reimbursement for relevant discharges. Those in the next decile received a 1% bonus, and those that did not meet a stated threshold by the third year of the project were to receive reduced payments.

Executives at Bon Secours Health System, based in Marriottsville, Maryland, described the project to the board of trustees and recommended that three or four of the system's high-performing hospitals participate. The board had other ideas. "They wanted to know why everyone shouldn't do this," remembers William Varani, M.D., vice president of quality for Bon Secours. "I told them that was a good idea, but some of our hospitals had weaker performance levels and needed time to improve. The board said, 'Let's make them improve. If they are part of this project and there's a chance they will be penalized for poor performance, won't they get better faster? Why wouldn't we want to do this with all of our hospitals?'" Management agreed that it made more sense for the hospitals with weaker performance to participate because it would give them more incentive to do what the high performers were already doing. Bon Secours joined the project as a system even though Premier explained there was a risk that the lowest 10% of the 20 hospitals involved would receive a penalty.

As a result of their work in the demonstration, the system's weaker hospitals have made great improvements. The initial median performance of all Bon Secours hospitals was at about 50%; the median performance in 2006 was at about 90%, and the system set the goal of 100% compliance with all the standards in all its hospitals by 2009. Management's initial overall corporate goal was to have all hospitals operating at above-the-median performance, but the board considered that goal to be too weak. The trustees didn't like the idea that their facilities would be only average. "They really pushed [for higher goals]," says Varani. "We were much more timid than our board." Thanks to the board's insistence, Bon Secours has had many success stories, including a challenged hospital in Baltimore that achieved a 68% increase in performance in the care of acute myocardial infarction.

process entails and why change is needed. Or you might choose to visit an area of your organization that has made great strides in quality or safety to congratulate staff members on their achievements and encourage progress elsewhere. The chair and members of the board at Sentara Healthcare like to visit hospitals within the system to see for themselves what is happening on the front lines. On one such visit, employees demonstrated a mnemonic that consisted of pointing to various parts of the body (eyes, mouth, ears, hand, arm) to remember five behavior-based safety expectations:

1. Eyes: Pay attention to detail, focusing attention on the task and decreasing skill-based errors.
2. Mouth: Communicate clearly, using repeat-backs and clarifying questions.
3. Ears: Have a questioning attitude, stopping actions when unsure and using the technique of "verify and validate."
4. Hand: Hand off effectively, using the "5P" checklist (patient or project, plan, purpose, problems, precautions).
5. Arm: Never leave your "wingman"; use peer checking and peer coaching when appropriate.

At the next board meeting, the chairman in turn demonstrated the mnemonic for the rest of the board. "Word of him doing that spread through the organization," recalls Gary Yates, M.D., senior vice president and chief medical officer, Sentara Healthcare. "It sent an important message to the company. The chairman of the board cared enough and was involved enough to see the demonstration, understand it, and take it back and explain it to the full board."

CASE STUDY: DANA-FARBER CANCER INSTITUTE

Dana-Farber Cancer Institute, Boston, is a teaching hospital affiliated with Harvard Medical School that specializes in cancer research and treatment. "We've had many successes, including the use of combination chemotherapy to treat childhood leukemia in the 1960s," says Saul N. Weingart, M.D., Ph.D., vice president for quality improvement and patient safety at Dana-Farber. "We've also seen some tragic failures, such as the accidental death of [a patient] in 1994 from a chemotherapy overdose that she received for an experimental breast cancer treatment." Rather than becoming demoralized after the sentinel event, Dana-Farber leadership acknowledged that mistakes occur and mobilized the organization—including the board of directors—to improve quality and patient safety. "The overdose affected our culture and the care we provide in an enduring way," says Weingart. "The board has led the effort to improve safety and quality since the 1990s."

Dana-Farber's board is made up of more than 100 members. A board-level quality committee comprised of 40 participants, 14 of whom are trustees, oversees quality and patient safety within the organization. "Members of the quality committee include trustees, senior leaders (including the chief nursing officer, chief operating officer, and chief medical officer), and representatives from the Adult and Pediatric Patient and Family Advisory Councils," says Weingart. The board quality committee regularly reports back to the full board regarding its progress. "The quality committee reviews critical incidents that occur in the institution, examining events that resulted in injury as well as near-miss errors, and focuses on the underlying systems problems that allowed these events to occur," says Weingart. "It's not about finger-pointing." In addition, the board tracks key safety indicators through a patient safety dashboard, including infection rates, adverse drug events, falls, and patient satisfaction measures. Finally, leadership updates the board on results from an annual safety culture survey and summarizes complaints or grievances from patients and family members.

Weingart notes that it takes a lot of work to support active and engaged board members. "If you ask for their advice, you need to act on it," says Weingart. "Working effectively with board members to drive improvement has been a valuable learning process for us."

Improving Medication Safety

The board quality committee has charged Dana-Farber leaders with conducting a prospective risk assessment each year to systematically identify and analyze vulnerabilities within the organization and to prioritize improvement initiatives. Board members, working with patients and staff, participate in the risk assessment. The recommendations are then reviewed by the board quality committee.

Dana-Farber's board quality committee has identified three major quality improvement initiatives that the board tracks closely:

1. A high-performance team training initiative across its ambulatory sites
2. Medication safety
3. Patient flow and experience

"At board meetings we spend half the time discussing and reviewing these three priority improvement areas," says Weingart. In addition, board subcommittees have been established to support leaders' efforts to implement an array of medication safety initiatives and the team training effort.

Medication safety, according to Weingart, "is an especially important project because so much of our patient care focuses on chemotherapy." Dana-Farber elicited feedback from staff members and invited the Institute for Safe Medication Practices to evaluate its medication processes. "We identified dozens of improvement opportunities related to medication safety," says Weingart. "The board members wanted to make sure we could adequately resource all of these projects." Under the guidance of the board quality committee, Dana-Farber provided resources such as the following to help accomplish this work:

- Hired a director of patient safety to help implement and track the projects
- Hired a medication safety officer in the pharmacy department
- Gained input from a process improvement specialist with a background in industrial engineering
- Introduced project management software to track projects over time

The board contributed to the effort to improve medication safety by forming a small subcommittee dedicated to that goal. "This subcommittee was formed to get closer to the action and also to allow executives to meet with board members who are invested in the process and who bring outside perspective and expertise," says Vincent O'Reilly, chair of the board quality committee.

Weingart adds, "For this effort, input from the board was extremely valuable. With so many new and ongoing projects related to medication safety, the board recognized that we needed to focus on project management. They helped us to organize these projects in a more sophisticated way."

Getting Involved with Joint Commission Accreditation

Dana-Farber's board members are informed of potential accreditation problem areas that may arise after conducting internal periodic performance reviews or after having an unannounced on-site survey. The board committee is kept apprised of compliance information that is reported back to The Joint Commission. "Board members also participate actively in the leadership session of the on-site surveys," says Weingart. For example, during the last Joint Commission survey, a board member on the quality committee explained to the surveyor how he applied his experience in running a large restaurant chain to help reduce patient wait times at Dana-Farber, says Janet Porter, executive vice president and chief operating officer. In addition, board members sit in to hear the surveyors' closing comments at the end of the survey. "The board thinks it is important to hear the findings of the surveyors directly," says O'Reilly.

Participating in Leadership WalkRounds

Senior leaders and trustees at Dana-Farber go on Leadership WalkRounds to visit clinical units throughout the organization at least once a month. "We think it's important to have a culture of safety that is transmitted from the board and senior management level to frontline staff, but we wanted to make it so that it was more than just words," says O'Reilly. These walkarounds allow leaders and trustees to understand issues or concerns that staff face when providing day-to-day care, and they help staff realize that the board members and leaders are interested and involved. "Leaders talk with frontline staff and ask about problems," says Weingart. "For example, a trustee asked nurses and managers at a satellite clinic about the quality of communication with the medical staff when physicians are off-site. She wanted to know how problems are sorted out collaboratively with the doctors and that there was a regular forum for doing so."

In regard to the satellite clinics, O'Reilly adds, "As Dana-Farber has evolved into a more geographically diverse entity, we wanted to make sure the clinics understood the culture of safety that is expected. When board members are included in the composition of people who come to visit a satellite clinic, it instantly conveys the value of a culture of safety. That is important to the board."

Gaining the Insights of Patients and Family Members

In addition to gaining staff input on patient safety and quality issues, Dana-Farber reaches out to patients for their insights on all aspects of the organization. To ensure that the patient's voice is heard, Dana-Farber created the Adult Patient and Family Advisory Council in 1998 and the Pediatric Patient and Family Advisory Council in 1999. Among other functions, the councils coordinate the appointment of patients and family members to more than 100 institutional committees and project teams. Patient representatives serve on the board quality committee. "Patients and family members bring a 'man-on-the-street' view of things," says Weingart. "They are a wonderful asset because they aren't shy about talking frankly to board members or senior executives. They can help us interpret patient satisfaction data and provide valuable insights on the feasibility and acceptability of proposed quality improvement projects. For example, we considered initiating a campaign for patients and family members to remind physicians and nurses to wash their hands. Some patient and family advisors worried that many patients would not feel comfortable in this role."

Holding Executives Accountable

The board holds Dana-Farber executives accountable for organization performance in ways such as the following:

- ➤ By requiring executives to follow up on outstanding and ongoing issues at board quality committee meetings
- ➤ By requesting improvement plans for items on the patient safety dashboard that do not meet benchmark performance

▶ By tying executive compensation to quality goals that are set by the board

Overall, Dana-Farber's board of directors provides the organization with insights from an "outside" perspective, access to resources, and motivation. "The executive team has a mature relationship with the board of directors," says Weingart. "We see them as a resource, helping us reach our goals rather than simply looking over our shoulders. They make sure we don't have tunnel vision—that we're not listening to ourselves alone, but also bringing in expert advice when necessary. The board honors and respects the work we do, but they also have an obligation to ensure that we do our jobs well."

Participating in Measurement and Improvement

As a board member, you do not participate in day-to-day measurement and improvement activities, but you are responsible for overseeing what those activities accomplish. Management brings organization goals and priorities for your review and approval. You can ask how well these fit into the organization's overall strategic plan, how specific goals were set (based on national averages, regulatory requirements, and so on), what resources will be necessary to reach those goals, and whether the goals are appropriate. If you don't have enough information to determine the answers to those questions, ask for more.

Many boards are taking the lead in quality and safety by urging management to aim higher than they originally planned. For example, executive leaders at Provena Saint Joseph Medical Center in Joliet, Illinois, shared best practices for emergency department turnaround times with their trustees. After presenting their numbers for indicators such as patients who left without being seen, patients who had been treated and "streeted" in less than three hours, and patients who had been treated and admitted to the hospital in less than four hours, the board asked what they were going to do to improve. "We explained to them that, on average, we were well above the national standards," remarks CEO Jeffrey Brickman. "They said, 'Okay, you've already done that. Now take a look at the averages and see if you can't further improve your overall average and go further above national best practice.'"

St. Vincent's Medical Center in Jacksonville, Florida, was an alpha site for Ascension Health's "Healthcare That Is Safe" initiative and was charged with identifying best practices for eliminating health care–associated pressure ulcers.[5] The board of directors supported this initiative by placing it on the board's agenda and making it one of a small number of strategic priorities. The board expressed interest in the hospital's progress and encouraged staff to reach for higher goals. "We had previously compared ourselves to national averages, and we always beat the national average," observes Wanda Gibbons, R.N., M.H.A., former vice president of patient care services and chief nursing officer at St. Vincent's. "With this project and Ascension's goals to eliminate all preventable injuries and death by 2008, we really changed our metric and said being better than the average isn't good enough. Our goal is zero. With the board's leadership and support of this initiative, we started seeing cultural changes. With any injury that is potentially avoidable, the right goal is zero."

Monitoring Performance

After your organization has set its goals, you need to know whether improvement efforts are meeting expectations, and if not, what can be done to facilitate progress. Perhaps work has stalled because more staff time is needed than was originally projected. Or the changes you originally planned may require a bigger cultural change than anticipated, meaning the goal will take longer to reach. In any case, you need to know what is happening with your organization's key initiatives. Boards may choose to monitor published quality measures from The Joint Commission (such as the National Patient Safety Goals or the ORYX® performance measures), CMS, the National Quality Forum, or the Agency for Healthcare Research and Quality.[6] In addition, boards may monitor organization-specific goals that need improvement (for example, reducing health care–associated infections or medication errors).[6]

Whether you are looking at trends in performance to set priorities or to monitor progress, you need information that is presented clearly and concisely in a format that is easy to use and understand. The same types of reports can be used for your full board and subcommittees (including the quality committee). You may want to urge management to send reports before meetings to allow you time to review the contents and formulate any questions or comments. This will save time at meetings by allowing you to focus your attention on areas that need it.

Dashboards. Many organizations use dashboards and scorecards to show their trustees how well they are performing in key areas. If you do not feel that you have sufficient or appropriate information to allow you to evaluate performance, or if the format(s) used for reports is not helpful, let management know so they can make changes.

There is no right or wrong way to organize a dashboard; however, when using the dashboard format, remember that it can become confusing if it contains too many indicators and metrics. Groups such as your board's quality committee may need more detail than your full board, so their dashboards may be more complex. But your entire board needs to see only areas important to your organization's specific quality and safety targets.

For example, organizations whose boards use dashboards with fewer measures (for example, 10 to 12 measures) but review them more frequently see better results in advancing patient safety and quality of care.[6,7] If individual committees feel that additional information is necessary, they can present it at the board meeting.

Reports. Although summary dashboards can be convenient, written reports that present important details about initiatives are also helpful for board members. You may find that you want to examine key topics more closely for prioritization or budgeting reviews, and a report that summarizes the relevant data in narrative form may be more useful than a general overview. For example, in addition to dashboards, St. Luke's Hospital in Cedar Rapids, Iowa, provides its board of trustees with a narrative summary of performance for each of its key indicators in the areas of mortality, patient satisfaction, patient safety, core measures, and emergency department treatment times.

Allocating Resources for Initiatives

Encouraging leaders and staff to strive for better outcomes and monitoring their progress is important, but you must be ready to back up your push for improved quality and safety with necessary resources. Staff members often complain that, with all their other duties, they do not have time to participate in improvement activities. Managers may need to order new software or computers to facilitate data collection and analysis. Or an improvement team may find that certain types of equipment, such as infusion pumps, need to be replaced with newer models that have better safety features. All these people will look to the board to supply the resources necessary for helping the organization provide better care.

After board members at Delnor-Community Hospital in Geneva, Illinois, adopted Project Zero (which aims to reduce the number of hospital-acquired infections), they stood behind this goal by providing enough resources to accomplish it. For example, when leaders suggested a method to further reduce *Clostridium difficile* infections by decontaminating those patient rooms with hydrogen peroxide vapor, board members gave them the green light to gather more information on purchasing this new technology. (For more information about how Delnor-Community Hospital's board gets involved in quality and patient safety, *see* the case study beginning below.)

CASE STUDY: DELNOR-COMMUNITY HOSPITAL

Delnor-Community Hospital, in Geneva, Illinois, has an influential and engaged board that has high expectations for the care provided at the hospital. However, as with most boards of health care organizations, this level of engagement in improving quality did not happen overnight. "Getting board members involved in quality improvement has been an evolutionary process," says John Hubbe, Pharm.D., J.D., vice president of medical and legal services, Delnor-Community Hospital, "but once board members knew what the best practices were and heard national speakers on quality, they wanted to know why we couldn't have that level of care at Delnor."

Melissa Coleman, board member and chair of the quality committee at Delnor, agrees, saying, "There was a point when we started talking about it and taking steps to make it a reality, and pretty soon it just became part of our everyday actions and decisions on the board." Furthermore, Coleman explained that the board members have a stake in the community and want Delnor to provide the highest quality of care. "The people we have on the board are from the community, and they are patients at Delnor along with their family and friends," says Coleman. "It's important to have the right people on the board who have a real interest in providing the best care for the larger community."

Educating Board Members

Education spurred Delnor's board to advocate for quality, and it continues to be a major priority. "Every year the board goes on an educational retreat for a day and a half. Quality has been one of the main themes for the last five years," says Coleman. Delnor also arranges for experts to meet with the board and share best practices. "We have had speakers meet with our board to discuss the responsibility of boards getting involved in quality," says Hubbe. The board also attends quarterly education sessions, which are separate from board meetings and focus on quality improvement issues. "All the board members take it upon themselves to read publications on quality improvement and stay up to date on the current issues in quality," says Coleman. "It's interesting to see the best practices in different hospitals. You find that one hospital may think an initiative is impossible, while another hospital takes the initiative on as a challenge and is successful."

Allocating Resources for Quality

Delnor's board members adopted Project Zero, which aims to reduce the number of hospital-acquired infections (including surgical site infections, *Clostridium difficile*, methicillin-resistant *Staphylococcus aureus*, and ventilator-associated pneumonia). Specifically, the board wanted to cut these infections in half by the end of 2010. "No patient should get an infection while they're staying in the hospital," says Hubbe. "We knew this goal was important, but the board understood that Project Zero had to be a long-term goal because it requires a great deal of strategy and resources to deploy," says Hubbe. Since 2006 Delnor has reduced the number of Project Zero infections by 75%. "When we met our goal of reducing these infections by half, we celebrated for a moment and then said, 'We can do more,'" says Coleman. Hubbe adds, "The board said, 'What don't you get about zero?' and we continued our work on reducing these infections."

After implementing evidence-based measures to reduce hospital-acquired infections, Delnor was delighted to see the infection rate drop as much as it did. But getting to zero is proving to be more difficult. "Because we're still seeing a few hospital-acquired *C. difficile* infections, we're looking into new technology for decontaminating an entire patient room with hydrogen peroxide vapor," says Hubbe. "Our board is committed to getting to zero, and they want us to gather more information about this product. It's an example where the board doesn't get into the day-to-day management, but they can allocate resources and recommend that we pursue further resources to be cutting-edge in reducing infections."

In addition to ad hoc requests for resources to achieve quality goals, management submits a formal budget for board approval annually. "Within the budget, we identify clinical quality highlights to show how we're allocating resources toward quality," says Hubbe. "Then the board understands how we're covering the quality issues financially."

Evaluating Performance Measurement

Delnor created a quality metrics dashboard with data on important safety measures related to Project Zero, acute myocardial infarction, heart failure, pneumonia, readmission rates, and mortality rates. As the chair of the quality committee, Coleman reviews the quality metrics dashboard with the board once a month. "It's not management giving the report," says Hubbe. "The board takes responsibility for understanding, measuring, and following through on these metrics."

Getting Involved with Joint Commission Accreditation

In addition to meeting with surveyors during the leadership conference at Joint Commission on-site surveys, board members at Delnor participate in root cause analyses (RCAs) for any sentinel events that occur within the organization. "We've had two members of the board-level quality committee participate on RCA teams to see the process firsthand," says Hubbe. "Although the board members are not trying to solve the problem, they are trying to understand how action plans are put in place to reduce the risk of an adverse event in the future. It's good for the board to get involved with the organization and see how we address system failures."

Participating on Hospital Committees

In addition, board members also regularly attend meetings with the medical staff executive committee, the credentialing committee, and the full medical staff, which meets on a quarterly basis. The chairman of the board, who regularly attends full medical staff meetings, will motivate physicians before the launch of new initiatives such as Project Zero. "He'll get in front of all the physicians and say, 'We may not be at the bedside with you, but in the boardroom we consider all the patients at Delnor to be our patients, too.' This sends a whole different signal about the expectations for quality care within the organization," says Hubbe.

Coleman describes how board members are familiarizing themselves with the credentialing process by going to credentialing committee meetings. "We're certainly not challenging their decisions at these meetings, but we are ultimately responsible for the process and need to understand how it's done. Then we have the assurance that we're appointing the right physicians at Delnor," says Coleman.

Gaining the Insights of Patients and Family Members

At every board-level quality committee meeting, a "patient experience" story is presented to highlight a measure on the quality metrics dashboard or to describe an incident that could be of concern. "Sometimes the patient or family member, the physician involved in the care of the patient, or an executive will tell the story," says Hubbe. "These patient stories give a face to the patient who acquired an infection under our care or to the patient who experienced a fall while in our hospital. When you do that, the medical jargon is taken away and the board members come face-to-face with the actual patient." Coleman adds, "We're looking at what happened, but also at how it affected the patient and his or her family. Then we want to know how leaders addressed this particular situation and what we are doing to make sure it doesn't happen again."

Holding Executives Accountable

Every year the board-level quality committee recommends quality measures to the compensation committee for setting organization goals, which are aligned with compensation for the CEO down through the management and frontline staff. "There is an expectation that you improve year after year no matter where you are," says Hubbe. "For example, we're at 94% for all core measures this year, so next year 94% is meeting expectations. In order to exceed expectations next year, you have to improve over 94%. The bar is set pretty high."

After meeting goals, the board congratulates leaders and staff members but then quickly refocuses their attention on further improvement. "We say, 'That's great, but we can do better,'" says Coleman. "And they prove us right all the time."

When the division of behavioral health services at Henry Ford Health System (Detroit) launched an initiative to eliminate suicides ("zero defects") among its 200,000 health plan members, the psychiatry department's board and the board's quality committee played a key role. They reviewed progress quarterly, provided encouragement to leaders and staff, and recognized accomplishments in written communications. They also undertook major philanthropic efforts to support the initiative; in particular, they raised substantial sums of money to support the development of critical information technology, including a Depression Care Web site for patients.[8]

In 2005 the board of directors at Provena Saint Joseph Medical Center began moving away from a focus on financial performance to a more balanced monthly review of indicators for patient safety, life safety, quality, and nursing. Based on the information they've received and the improvements they've supported, the trustees have approved resources for staff to work on introducing bar coding into the medication process, for electronic monitoring in the intensive care unit, and to increase nurse staffing by allocating $2.7 million for this purpose.

When Iowa Health System's board members requested a multiyear proposal for systemwide safety initiatives in 2006, they also made it known that they were ready to back those initiatives with resources. "They asked, 'What is it going to take? What resources do you need?'" says Kent Bottles, M.D., the system's former vice president and chief medical officer. "We also see evidence of boards in individual hospitals backing [quality efforts]. Discussion of falls and how to prevent them has gotten fairly detailed at some of the board meetings. The board in Des Moines, for example, reviews the fall data and has some physician board members who have become very vocal about this because they're so grateful that they're not getting calls anymore saying their patients have fallen. Their numbers are quite low compared to what they used to be, and they talk about what they're doing to make this difference, such as using different beds, different bed alarms, and so on. When we have those discussions and see those resources being distributed, there's a clear-cut connection."

Holding Management Accountable for Change

Because the governing body is responsible for the performance of an entire organization, it makes sense that the CEO and other senior leaders should be held responsible for helping the organization meet its performance goals. Some executives may feel that such accountability is unfair, given that their ability to achieve positive results depends in part on how much support they receive from the board. If trustees set unrealistic goals or refuse to provide the resources necessary to achieve goals, there is little chance that the CEO can effect required changes. However, the emphasis of accountability is on gaining executive commitment to help the organization deliver the best health care possible.

One way to promote accountability is to incorporate quality and safety goals into senior leaders' or even midlevel managers' annual performance evaluations. These goals will differ from one organization and setting to another, but they should align with the overall strategic goals the board has approved. For example, goals may address clinical indicators such as ORYX core measures, patient satisfaction, compliance with National Patient Safety Goals, or provision of necessary staffing. Even though money can provide leaders with the incentive to reach quality improvement goals, a recent survey of chairpersons found that only 44% include quality of care in their two most important criteria for evaluating the CEO's performance.[1]

However, an Integrated Healthcare Strategies survey found that nearly 83% of organizations provide incentive plans to senior executives (including the CEO).[6] Furthermore, this survey also noted that 58% of organizations provide incentive plans to directors, 47% provide incentives to physicians employed by the organization, 38% to service-line managers, 34% to middle managers, and 27% to frontline employees.[6]

Iowa Health System board members drew on clinical quality and safety measures to develop an incentive program for its hospital CEOs. Including patient safety metrics in the CEO compensation "report card" has helped to align the system and local facility strategic goals and gives senior leaders across the system an incentive to share information on improvement efforts. Maulik S. Joshi and Stephen C. Hines, who interviewed CEOs and board chairpersons from 30 hospitals in a study on the role of hospital governance in quality, advise that linking CEO compensation with quality is becoming the norm—that hospital boards that do not already incentivize quality through CEO compensation should consider doing so.[9]

If you have never before linked organization safety and quality of care to executive performance, you may need to introduce changes to bonus payments by degrees. As your organization becomes more focused on quality and safety, leaders will be more likely to agree with and even promote the move away from finance-based achievement. Several years ago, 25% of variable compensation for the top 100 executives within Sentara Healthcare was based on quality and patient safety. However, with management recommendations and board support, that amount has increased to 40%.

For quality and safety initiatives to succeed, they need to be as fully integrated into the organization's culture and operations as fiscal prudence and operational excellence. William F. Jessee, M.D., F.A.C.M.P.E, F.A.C.P.M., former chair of the board of directors of Exempla Health System (Denver), states, "Economic incentives for everyone in the organization must be aligned with quality and safety as well as with margins and market share. In the organization, senior executives have explicit quality and safety goals included as a significant part of their incentive compensation formula. Contracts with physicians for medical director services or for hospital-based physician services similarly include quality and safety performance targets and financial incentives for achieving those targets." Bonus incentives for frontline employees at Exempla are based on patient satisfaction and will be expanded to include appropriate quality and safety goals. Jessee emphasizes that "it all starts with the board. If the board doesn't set the expectation that quality and safety are as important to it as financial performance, how can management and medical staff be expected to make it a priority?"

Boards can follow Exempla's example in tying all employees' performance to quality improvement. An important step is assessing each employee's ability to meet patient safety and quality goals at annual performance reviews. For example, Sentara Healthcare created the Performance Plus program, wherein employees receive financial compensation when the organization meets certain goals, at least 50% of which are related to quality and patient safety.[6]

Addressing Quality and Safety in Board Meetings

Boards have a limited amount of time to spend on any one topic, so quality and safety must be scheduled on the agenda to ensure that they receive appropriate attention. If you have a quality subcommittee (or any group dedicated to quality and safety), its members can help disseminate the most important information to the full board. At Exempla, as Jessee relates, the board's quality committee operates much like the finance committee: "The quality committee reviews quality performance data from our three hospitals, evaluates responses to sentinel events, oversees medical staff credentialing and privileges recommendations, monitors public reporting of quality data, and reports regularly to the full board."

Jessee continues, "Consistency is encouraged in care processes and policies among the three hospitals and learnings from one are used to stimulate improvements in the others." Like the finance committee, the quality committee "not only reports to the full board but also helps the board focus its discussions on important opportunities to improve safety and quality across the system." The quality committee, adds Jessee, "has played an important role in improving the board's involvement and engagement in quality and safety. And it has also given the board renewed assurance that it is exercising the same fiduciary responsibility for the quality and safety of care as it does for the financial performance of the hospitals."

As discussed earlier, dashboards and focused reports can keep board members current on how improvement initiatives are progressing and where attention and resources need to be focused. You need enough time not only for reporting but also for asking questions about and discussing changes in performance. If a topic or project in which you are particularly interested is not covered, inquire about it.

Administration and the quality committee have to prioritize what they present within the time constraints they're given. If they know about your concerns, they can arrange to update you after the meeting or bring the information to the next one.

If your board has traditionally given most of its time to fiscal matters, putting quality and safety at the top of your agenda can send a clear message to both trustees and administration that your priorities have shifted. The Institute for Healthcare Improvement recommends that boards spend more than 25% of their meeting time on quality and safety issues.[10]

Several years ago, the board of trustees at Johns Hopkins moved quality to the top of its agenda and finances to the bottom. Members receive updates from administration and reports from the quality committee before discussing any other business. "Doing something relatively small like putting quality at the top of the agenda makes a big difference along the way," notes Richard Davis. "It not only sends a clear message, it causes some creative tension throughout the organization because now everyone knows [quality and safety are] a high-level priority." Nor are trustees satisfied to simply listen to presentations and move on. "Our board members are very astute and will ask difficult and challenging questions, as they should," says Davis. Davis often brings staff members who have been working on improvement projects to board meetings; this serves the dual purpose of bringing the work to the board in a more personal way and of giving frontline workers some recognition.

You may want to ask the administration to include patients and family members in the quality section of your agenda as well. Patients and family members can give you a fresh perspective on how your organization delivers care and can provide a "human face" to the care represented by the performance data you routinely review. It has been proposed that boards talk with at least one patient or family member about any serious harm the patient may have encountered at the organization.[10]

Patient opinions can also be brought to the table by board members or administrators who have worked directly with patients. For example, Dana-Farber Cancer Institute's patient/family organizations are consulted on many initiatives to improve care. These organizations have representation on the hospital's joint quality committee, which also includes trustees. Their opinions are solicited and considered on topics ranging from the planning of new buildings to processes for dealing with

Chapter 3

immunocompromised patients in the emergency department. At one board-level quality committee meeting, Maureen Connor, R.N., M.P.H., former vice president for quality improvement and risk management, presented a close call that had been identified by a patient. During the ensuing discussion, committee members discussed the role of patients in identifying and reporting medical errors. The patient members explained how although some patients can play a role in error identification, the ultimate responsibility should rest with clinicians and that many patients have no desire to assume this responsibility. Connor states, "It reminded me of leadership's need to remain sensitive to patient concerns when promoting initiatives around patient empowerment. I left this particular meeting wondering how such discussions can possibly take place without a patient at the table." (For more information about how Dana-Farber involves patients in board meetings, *see* the case study on pages 80–85.)

The Next Step

Patience, commitment, enthusiasm, motivation, and the willingness to learn—these are some of the qualities you need as you push your organization toward safer, higher-quality care. You may encounter resistance to change from senior leaders or staff. You may find that your entire organization, including certain board members, requires additional training in quality concepts, best practices, and national safety recommendations. You may need to make difficult decisions regarding the distribution of resources to accomplish strategic quality goals. All these challenges are a normal part of the journey toward your ultimate goal of providing the safest, highest-quality care possible.

As a board member, you have many opportunities to lead by example. The interest you and your fellow trustees show for quality and safety issues will be mirrored in the efforts of senior leaders and staff to improve processes and systems. Whether you are demanding higher goals for quality initiatives, encouraging transparency in reporting, or celebrating the successes of improvement teams, you are showing both internal and external stakeholders that quality and safety are top priorities in your organization. "The thing I try to tell other boards and board chairmen is that anybody can pay attention," says Lee Carter. "You don't have to be a surgeon or a nurse to pay attention, and that really is the role of the board."

Are you ready to take on the challenge?

References

1. Jha A., Epstein A.: Hospital governance and the quality of care. *Health Aff (Millwood)* 29: 182–187, Jan.–Feb. 2010.
2. Jiang H.J., Bass K., Fraser I.: Board oversight of quality: Any differences in process of care and mortality? *J Healthc Manag* 54:15–29, Jan.–Feb. 2009.
3. Frankel A., et al.: Patient Safety Leadership WalkRounds™. *Jt Comm J Qual Saf* 29:16–26, Jan. 2003.
4. Frankel A., et al.: Patient Safety Leadership WalkRounds at Partners Healthcare: Learning from implementation. In Frankel A.S. (ed.): *Strategies for Building a Hospitalwide Culture of Safety.* Oakbrook Terrace, IL: Joint Commission Resources, 2006, pp. 127–141.
5. Gibbons W., et al.: Eliminating facility-acquired pressure ulcers in Ascension Health. *Jt Comm J Qual Patient Saf* 32:488–496, Sep. 2006.
6. ECRI Institute: Incentives for patient safety: Holding healthcare executives accountable. *Risk Management Reporter* 27:1–10, Aug. 2008.
7. Miller T.E., Gutmann V.L.: Changing expectations for board oversight of healthcare quality: The emerging paradigm. *J Health Life Sci Law* 2:31, 33, Jul. 2009.
8. Coffey C.E.: Building a system of perfect depression care in behavioral health. *Jt Comm J Qual Patient Saf* 33:193–199, Apr. 2007.
9. Joshi M.S., Hines S.C.: Getting the board on board: Engaging hospital boards in quality and patient safety. *Jt Comm J Qual Patient Saf* 32:179–187, Apr. 2006.
10. Institute for Healthcare Improvement: *Getting Started Kit: Governance Leadership How-to Guide* (Get Boards on Board). http://www.ihi.org/IHI/Programs/Campaign/BoardsonBoard.htm (accessed Feb. 7, 2011).

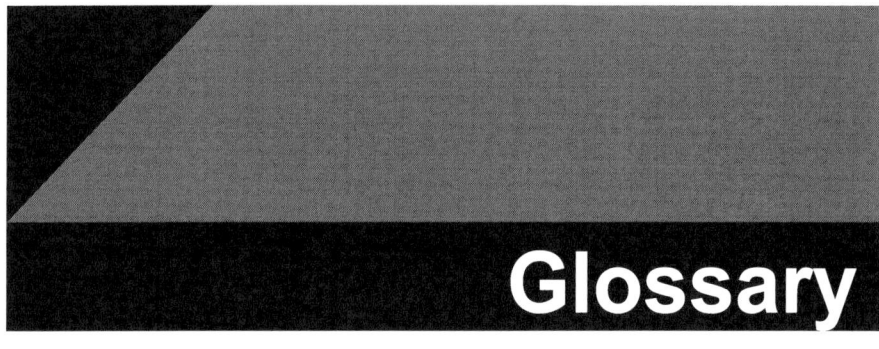

Glossary

accreditation Determination by The Joint Commission that an eligible organization complies with applicable Joint Commission accreditation requirements.

accreditation manual A Joint Commission publication consisting of policies, procedures, and accreditation requirements relating to ambulatory care, office-based surgery, behavioral health care, critical access hospital, home care, hospital services, long term care, and pathology and clinical laboratory services. Organizations should use the manual that contains the set of accreditation requirements most appropriate to their primary focus or mission.

adverse drug event An injury resulting from a medical intervention related to a medication, including harm from a drug reaction or a medication error.

best practices Clinical, scientific, or professional practices that are recognized by a majority of professionals in a particular field. These practices are typically evidence based and consensus driven.

board The individual(s), group, or agency that has ultimate authority and responsibility for establishing policy, maintaining quality of care, and providing for organization management and planning. Other names for this group include *governance, board of trustees, board of governors, board of commissioners,* and *governing body.*

clinical/service groups (CSGs) Groups of patients, residents, or individuals served and/or services in distinct, clinical populations on whom data are collected. Tracers for patients, residents, or individuals served are selected according to CSGs.

close call Any variation during the provision of care, treatment, or services that did not affect an outcome but for which a recurrence carries a significant risk of an adverse outcome. Also known as a near miss, a close call is a sentinel event by definition but is not subject to review by The Joint Commission under its Sentinel Event Policy.

credentialing The process of obtaining, verifying, and assessing the qualifications of a practitioner to provide care or services in or for a health care organization.

evidence-based guidelines Guidelines that have been scientifically developed based on recent literature review and that are consensus driven.

health care–associated infection An infection acquired during the course of receiving medical care. The infection may or may not have resulted from the care, treatment, or services received.

The Joint Commission An independent, not-for-profit organization, The Joint Commission is dedicated to improving the safety and quality of health care through standards development, public policy initiatives, accreditation, and certification. The Joint Commission accredits and certifies more than 18,000 health care organizations and programs in the United States.

leader An individual who sets expectations, develops plans, and implements procedures to assess and improve the quality of the organization's governance, management, and clinical and support functions and processes. At a minimum, leaders include members of the governing body and medical staff, the chief executive officer and other senior managers, the nurse executive, clinical leaders, and staff members in leadership positions.

leadership group Individuals in senior positions with clearly defined, unique responsibilities. These might include governance, management, medical staff, and clinical staff. Not every organization will have all these groups, and an individual may be a member of more than one group.

medical staff The group of all licensed independent practitioners and other practitioners privileged through the organized medical staff process that is subject to the medical staff bylaws. This group may include others, such as retired practitioners who no longer practice in the organization but who wish to continue their membership in the group, courtesy staff, scientific staff, and so on.

medication error A preventable event that may cause or lead to inappropriate medication use or patient harm while the medication is in the control of the health care professional, patient, or consumer. Such events may be related to professional practice, health care products, procedures, and systems, including prescribing; order communication; product labeling, packaging, and nomenclature; compounding; dispensing; distribution; administration; education; monitoring; and use.

performance improvement Data collection and analysis to assess the organization's progress on a specified process or outcome.

performance measurement system A method of gauging organization performance that facilitates improvement through the collection of data and information and the dissemination of process and/or outcome measures over time.

priority focus areas (PFAs) A process, system, or structure in a health care organization that significantly affects the quality and safety of care. PFAs guide a surveyor in assessing standards compliance in relation to individual tracer activity.

root cause analysis (RCA) A process for identifying basic or causal factor(s) underlying variation in performance, including the occurrence or possible occurrence of a sentinel event.

safety The degree to which an intervention (for example, use of a drug or a procedure) in the care environment is free of risk for a patient and other persons, including health care practitioners. Safety risks may arise from the performance of tasks, from the structure of the physical environment, or from situations beyond the organization's control (such as weather).

sentinel event An unexpected occurrence involving death or serious physical or psychological injury or risk thereof. Serious injury specifically includes loss of limb or function. The phrase "or risk thereof" includes any process variation for which a recurrence would carry a significant chance of a serious adverse outcome.

standard A principle of patient safety and quality of care that a well-run organization meets. A standard defines the performance expectations, structures, or processes required to enhance the quality of care, treatment, or services.

tracer methodology A process surveyors use on site to analyze an organization's systems, with particular attention to identified priority focus areas, by following an individual patient, resident, or individual served through the organization's care process in the sequence experienced by each individual. Depending on the setting, this process may require surveyors to visit multiple care programs and services within an organization or within a single program or service to "trace" the care rendered.

Index

A

Abduction, 55
Accountability measures, 4, 51–52
Accountable care organizations, 3
Accreditation. *See also* Standards
  board's role in, 47, 83, 90
  continuous improvement and, 35, 36
  goal of, 53
  Joint Commission programs and services related to, 4, 33
  Medicare program eligibility and, 35
  number of accredited health care providers, 34
  Priority Focus Process, 45–47, 52, 53
  revision of process for, 36
  Strategic Surveillance System (S3), 4, 52–53
  tracer methodology, 48–49
  types of organizations eligible for, 34
  unannounced surveys, 47–48
Accreditation Council for Graduate Medical Education, 20
Accreditation status, 4
Adult Patient and Family Advisory Council, 84
Advancing Effective Communication, Cultural Competence, and Patient- and Family-Centered Care (Joint Commission), 20
Adverse events
  accountability measures, 51
  adverse drug events
    computerized monitoring of, 25
    prevention of, 12
  CMS reporting system, 6
  patient role in avoidance of, 14–15, 59–60
  prevention of, 12
  proactive approach to prevention of, 17–21
  reporting of, 16–17
  reporting of, requirement for, 13
  response to, standard on, 35
  serious reportable events, 6, 13
Affordable Health Care Act, 2–3
Agency for Healthcare Research and Quality
  IHI initiatives, endorsement of, 11
  monitoring performance through measures from, 86
  quality and safety study by, v–vi
  quality measures, development of, 3
  20 Tips to Help Prevent Medical Errors, 15
Aims for Improvement (Institute of Medicine), 9
Air embolism, 8
Alcohol core measure set, 50
All-hazards command structure, 28
American Board of Medical Specialties, 20
American College of Physicians, 11
American Medical Association, 11
Anticoagulation therapy, 57
Application for accreditation, 45
Arm, 80
Ascension Health, "Healthcare That Is Safer" initiative, 86
Assault, 16
Asthma, children's
  core measure set on, 50
  process-of-care measure on, 7
Audits, internal and external, 14
Australia, 1
Automated dispensing machines, 25

B

Bacterial infections, 27
Banner Health case study, 74, 75–77
Bar-coding technology, 25
Behavior-based safety expectations, 80
Behaviors, disruptive and inappropriate, 42
Bermuda, 1
Bioterrorism treats, 26
Blood incompatibility issues, 8, 55
Blood management core measure set, 50
Board
    accountability of, 13–14, 77, 84–85, 91–92, 93–95
    accreditation process, role in, 47, 83, 90
    education and training of, vi, 74–75, 76, 89
    effectiveness of, 36
    familiarity with quality and safety issues, 1, 15, 71
    independence of board members, 14
    involvement in quality and safety improvements, vi, 11, 12, 13, 71–74, 85–88, 90, 97–98
    leadership standards and responsibilities of, 36, 37–44
    meetings of, discussions about quality issues at, 72, 95–97
    modeling good communication techniques, 20–21
    quality committees and subcommittees, vi, 72, 73, 95–96
    questions board members should ask themselves, vii
    responsibility for quality and safety, v–vi, 36, 38–39, 71–72, 97–98
Bon Secours Health System quality incentive demonstration participation, 79
Brigham and Women's Hospital Patient Safety Leadership WalkRounds, 77
Budget and finance, responsibility for, 36
Bundled payments, 3

C

California HealthCare Foundation, 11
Canada, 1
Care, treatment, and services
    complaints or concerns about, process for reporting, 53–54
    coordination of care, 9
    coordination of care at transitions, 49
    delay in treatment, 16
    methods and techniques, advances in, 9
    NQF safe practices, 6
    patient involvement in, 14–15, 59–60, 97
    performance reports on, vi
    prices for items and services, availability of, 3
    reimbursements for, v
    spending on, 1
Case studies and examples
    Banner Health, 74, 75–77
    Bon Secours Health System quality incentive demonstration participation, 79
    Brigham and Women's Hospital Patient Safety Leadership WalkRounds, 77
    Dana-Farber Cancer Institute
        case study, 78, 80–85
        quality committee, patient and family participants on, 96–97
    Delnor-Community Hospital, 88–92
    Exempla Health System
        compensation for employees, basis for, 94–95
        quality committee, 95
    Henry Ford Health System suicide prevention initiative, 92
    Iowa Health System
        incentive program for CEO compensation, 94
        quality improvement initiatives, 74–75
        resources for improvement activities, 92–93
    Johns Hopkins Hospital
        board meeting discussions about quality and safety issues, 96
        executive rounding program, 78

Index

Provena Saint Joseph Medical Center
  emergency department initiative, 85
  performance improvement initiatives, 92
St. Luke's Hospital performance monitoring dashboards and reports, 87
St. Vincent's Medical Center "Healthcare That Is Safer" initiative, 86
Sentara Healthcare
  compensation for employees, basis for, 94, 95
  Performance Plus program, 95
  quality subcommittee policy, 72
  walkarounds program, 80
Center for Medicare and Medicaid Innovation, 3
Center for Transforming Healthcare
  establishment of, 4, 58
  participants of, 33
  purpose and goals of, 4–5, 33, 58
  quality solutions developed by, 5, 22–23
  RPI methods use by, 5, 58
  targeted solutions development, 23, 33
  Targeted Solutions Tool, 5, 23, 27, 58
Centers for Disease Control and Prevention (CDC)
  hand hygiene guidelines, compliance with, 57
  health care–associated infections, 26, 27
Centers for Medicare & Medicaid Services
  adverse events, reporting of to, 6
  bundled payments, 3
  Center for Medicare and Medicaid Innovation, 3
  Conditions of Participation and accreditation, 35
  hospital-acquired conditions, nonreimbursable, 6–7
  hospital-acquired conditions, penalties for, 3
  Hospital Compare, 3, 7
  Hospital Consumer Assessment of Healthcare Providers and Systems, 7, 45
  IHI initiatives, endorsement of, 11
  incentive payments program, 51
  Medicare and Medicaid payments, decrease in, 2, 4
  Medicare program eligibility and Joint Commission accreditation, 35
  Medicare Severity-Diagnosis Related Group, 3
  monitoring performance through measures from, 86
  National Hospital Inpatient Quality Measures, 50
  payment system, health care reform and, 3
  Premier Hospital Quality Incentive Demonstration, 79
  quality and safety, role in, 6
  quality measures, development of, 3
  reimbursements from, 6
  Speak Up program, 59
Central line infections
  causes of, 27
  as nonreimbursable hospital-acquired condition, 8
  prevention of, 12, 57
Certification. *See also* Standards
  continuous improvement and, 35
  disease-specific care programs, 34–35
  health care staffing services, 34
  Joint Commission programs and services related to, 33
Change management, 5
Charity care, qualifications for, 3
Chronic conditions, care for patients with, 9
Clinical/service groups, 45–46, 53
Close calls
  definition of, 16
  as opportunities to correct problems, 18
  reporting errors related to, 16
Clostridium difficile infections, 88, 89–90, 91
Code of conduct, 42
Collaborative relationships, 18, 20, 24
Committee on the Quality of Health Care in America (Institute of Medicine), 7

Committees
    hospital committees, participation on, 91
    patient and family member representatives on, 84, 96–97
    quality committees and subcommittees, vi, 72, 73, 95–96
Communication
    culture of safety and quality and, 20
    effective communication, 19–21, 43, 57
    between leaders, 40–41
    modeling good communication techniques, 20–21
    National Patient Safety Goal on, 57
    with patients and family members, 19–20, 43
    safety and quality information, communication of (LD.03.04.01), 43
    between staff members, 20–21
    standard related to, 19
    training on methods for, 20
Community health needs
    assessment of, 3
    report on activities to meet, 3
Communitywide emergencies, planning for, 28
Complaints about care, process for reporting, 53–54
Computerized decision support systems, 25, 26
Computerized provider order entry, 25, 26
Concerns about care, process for reporting, 53–54
Conflicts among leadership groups (LD.02.04.01), 41
Conflicts of interest, 14, 40
Congestive heart failure, readmissions for, 12
Critical test results
    computerized notification of, 25
    timely reporting of, 57
Crossing the Quality Chasm (Institute of Medicine), 9–10
Cultural barriers, 19
Culture of safety and quality
    communication and, 20
    creation of, 17–18
    promotion of, 73–75, 78, 80
    standard related to, 18, 41–42

D

Dana-Farber Cancer Institute
    case study, 78, 80–85
    quality committee, patient and family participants on, 96–97
Dashboards, vi, 72, 87
Data and information use in decision making (LD.03.02.01), 42–43
Data use system tracer, 49
Decision support systems, computerized, 25, 26
Deep vein thrombosis, 8
Delnor-Community Hospital case study, 88–92
Depression Care Web site, 92
Disease-specific care programs, 34–35
Disruptive behaviors, 42
Drug-resistant organisms, 26, 57

E

Early Survey Policy, 48
Ears, 80
Electronic medical records, 25
Emergency management
    all-hazards command structure, 28
    focus of, 28
    plan for, 28
Environmental safety, 27
Errors
    attention given to, 2
    causes of, 16
    culture of safety and quality and reporting of, 17–18
    deaths from, 7
    Institute of Medicine report on, 7, 9
    patient role in avoidance of, 14–15, 59–60, 97

proactive approach to prevention of,
17–21
punitive environment and reporting of, 18
reporting of, 16–17
sentinel events compared to, 16
Ethics code, 14
Evidence-based practices
health care–associated infections, prevention of, 57
IHI initiatives to promote, 12
promotion of use of, 6
readmission rates, reduction of, 2
Exempla Health System
compensation for employees, basis for, 94–95
quality committee, 95
Eyes, 80

F

Falls
as nonreimbursable hospital-acquired condition, 8
prevention initiatives, 93
as sentinel event, 16
staffing shortages and, 23
Family members
committees, participation on, 84, 96–97
communication with, 19–20, 43
insight about quality and safety issues through, 91, 96–97
Finance and budget, responsibility for, 36
Financial information
audits, internal and external, 14
statements and information, accuracy of, 14
5 Million Lives Campaign (IHI), 11, 12
Fluoroscopy, prolonged, 55
Foreign object retained after surgery, 8, 16, 55

G

Germany, 1
Glossary, 99–102
Glycemic control, poor, 8
Governing body, v. *See also* Board

H

H1N1 influenza, 26
Hand, 80
Hand hygiene
compliance with, quality solution for, 5
compliance with guidelines on, 57
compliance with hand hygiene practices, 27
infection prevention and control and, 27
targeted solutions for, 27, 58
Hand-off communication
definition of, 22
National Patient Safety Goal on, 22, 23
prevalence of errors during, 22
quality solutions for, 5, 22–23
targeted solutions for, 23, 58
Health care–associated infections. *See also* Hospital-acquired conditions
deaths from, 26
drug-resistant organisms, 26, 57
ineffective infection prevention and control practices and, 27
National Patient Safety Goal on, 57
prevalence of, 26
prevention of, 57
Project Zero, 88, 89–90, 91
reporting of, 13
staffing shortages and, 23
Health care industry
accountability for care, 12–14
challenges for, 9–10, 71
conflicts of interest, 14, 40
ethics code, 14
goals of, 1–2
national health care reform legislation, v, 2–4
President's Advisory Commission on

107

Consumer Protection and Quality in the
  Health Care Industry, 5
  Sarbanes-Oxley Act and, 14
Health care professionals. *See* Physicians
  and health care professionals
Health care reform
  challenges of, 1–2
  national health care reform legislation, v,
    2–4
Health care staffing services, 34
"Healthcare That Is Safer" initiative
  (Ascension Health), 86
Health literacy issues, 19
Heart attack
  aspirin for patients with, 51
  core measure set on, 49
  outcomes-of-care measure on, 7
  prevention of, 12
  process-of-care measure on, 7
Heart failure
  core measure set on, 49
  left ventricular systolic function assessment, 52
  non-accountability measures, 52
  outcomes-of-care measure on, 7
  process-of-care measure on, 7
Henry Ford Health System suicide prevention initiative, 92
Hepatitis, 26
Herbal medications, 25
Hierarchical cultures, 18
High-alert medications, reduction of harm from, 12
HIV, 26
Homicide, 16
Hospital-acquired conditions. *See also*
    Health care–associated infections
  nonreimbursable, 6–7, 8
  penalties for, 3
  quality data on, 7
Hospital Compare, 3, 7
*Hospital Consumer Assessment of
  Healthcare Providers and Systems*, 7,
  45

Hospital Quality and Safety Survey (Leapfrog
  Group), 10–11
Hospitals
  imaging tests for outpatients, 7
  performance data, reporting of, 7
  prices for items and services, availability
    of, 3
  readmission for congestive heart failure
    patients, 12
  readmission rates
    interventions to decrease, 2
    outcomes-of-care measure on, 7
    reduced payments for higher-than-
      expected rates, 3
  tax-exempt status, activities to maintain, 3
Hydrogen peroxide vapor, decontamination
  with, 88, 89–90

I

IHI. *See* Institute for Healthcare Improvement
  (IHI)
Imaging tests for outpatients, 7
Incident command system, 28
Individual-based system tracers, 49
Individual tracer activities, 48–49
Infants
  discharge to wrong family, 55
  hyperbilirubinemia, 55
  mortality rates, 1
  perinatal care core measure set, 50
  perinatal death/loss of function, 16, 55
Infection prevention and control
  health care–associated infections
    deaths from, 26
    drug-resistant organisms, 26, 57
    ineffective infection prevention and
      control practices and, 27
    National Patient Safety Goal on, 57
    prevalence of, 26
    prevention of, 57
    Project Zero, 88, 89–90, 91
    reporting of, 13
    staffing shortages and, 23

Index

plan for, 26–27
surgical site infections
  causes of, 27
  as nonreimbursable hospital-acquired condition, 8
  prevention of, 12, 57
  quality solution for, 5
  targeted solutions for, 58
system tracer, infection control, 49
threat from infections, 26
Infection Prevention and Control (IC) standards, 27
Influenza outbreaks, 26, 27
Influenza vaccinations, 27, 51
Initial surveys, 48
Institute for Healthcare Improvement (IHI)
  100,000 Lives Campaign, 11, 12
  5 Million Lives Campaign, 11, 12
  board meeting discussions about quality and safety issues, 96
Institute of Medicine
  Aims for Improvement, 9
  Committee on the Quality of Health Care in America, 7
  Crossing the Quality Chasm, 9–10
  To Err Is Human, 7, 9, 10, 14–15
Insurance
  insured Americans, increase in, v, 2, 4
  requirement to enroll in, 2
  uninsured Americans, number of, 1
Integrated Healthcare Strategies survey, 93–94
Intensive care unit measures, 52
Internal Revenue Service, 3
Iowa Health System
  incentive program for CEO compensation, 94
  quality improvement initiatives, 74–75
  resources for improvement activities, 92–93

J

JCI (Joint Commission International), 33
JCR (Joint Commission Resources), 33, 60
Johns Hopkins Hospital
  board meeting discussions about quality and safety issues, 96
  executive rounding program, 78
Joint Commission
  Advancing Effective Communication, Cultural Competence, and Patient- and Family-Centered Care, 20
  Center for Transforming Healthcare (*see* Center for Transforming Healthcare)
  early name of, 33
  establishment of, 33
  IHI initiatives, endorsement of, 11
  mission of, 4, 33
  National Hospital Inpatient Quality Measures, 50
  Office of Quality Monitoring, 53–54
  programs and services of, 4
  Quality Monitoring System database, 45
  Smart Parent's Guide to Getting Your Kids Through Checkups, Illnesses, and Accidents, 60
  Speak Up, 15, 59
  Speak Up program, 59
  YOU: The Smart Patient, 15, 59–60
Joint Commission Connect extranet site
  ORYX Performance Measurement Report access, 51
  Priority Focus Process Report access, 46
  S3 reports access, 53
  Targeted Solutions Tool, access to, 5
Joint Commission International (JCI), 33
Joint Commission Resources (JCR), 33, 60

L

Labeling medications, medication containers, and solutions, 57
Language barriers, 19
Latent system failures, 16–17

Leadership
- accountability of, 77, 84–85, 91–92, 93–95
- communication between leaders, 40–41
- compensation for CEOs, basis for, 14, 94
- conflicts among leadership groups, 41
- modeling good communication techniques, 20–21
- quality improvement and CEO evaluation, vi, 73, 93–95
- responsibility for, 36
- training of on quality and safety principles and measures, 74
- walkarounds, 77–78, 80, 83–84

Leadership (LD) standards
- board's responsibilities and, 36, 37–44
- communication between leaders (LD.02.03.01), 40–41
- conflicts among leadership groups (LD.02.04.01), 41
- conflicts of interest (LD.02.02.01), 40
- culture of safety and quality (LD.03.01.01), 41–42
- data and information use in decision making (LD.03.02.01), 42–43
- focus of, 36
- knowledge of leaders (LD.01.07.01), 39
- leadership structure (LD.01.01.01), 37
- performance improvement activities (LD.03.05.01), 44
- planning activities to support safety and quality (LD.03.03.01), 43
- responsibilities of leaders (LD.01.02.01), 37–38
- revision of, 36
- safety and quality, accountability for (LD.01.03.01), 38–39
- safety and quality, improvement of (LD.03.06.01), 44
- safety and quality information, communication of (LD.03.04.01), 43

Leadership session, 83
Lean Six Sigma, 5, 58
Lean Thinking, 5, 22

Leapfrog Group, 10–11
- Hospital Quality and Safety Survey, 10–11
- Leapfrog Hospital Rewards Program, 10
- Rewarding Results initiative, 11

Liability claims, resolution of, 2
Look-alike/sound-alike drugs, 25

M

Mail-order pharmacies, 25
Maternal deaths, 56
Medicaid. *See* Centers for Medicare & Medicaid Services
Medical equipment, cleaning and disinfection of, 27
Medical imaging tests for outpatients, 7
Medicare. *See* Centers for Medicare & Medicaid Services
Medicare Severity-Diagnosis Related Group, 3
Medications
- adverse drug events, prevention of, 12
- errors
  - MEDMARX database on, 25
  - prevalence of, 24
  - as sentinel event, 16
  - staffing shortages and, 23
  - technology to prevent, 25–26
- herbal medications, 25
- high-alert medications, reduction of harm from, 12
- look-alike/sound-alike drugs, 25
- management of
  - challenges of, 24–25
  - processes for, 24
  - system tracer, medication management, 49
  - technology for, 25–26
- medication reconciliation process, 12, 25, 57
- National Patient Safety Goal on, 57
- over-the-counter medications, 25
- safety of
  - anticoagulation therapy, 57

Index

improvement of, 81–83
labeling medications, medication containers, and solutions, 57
verbal orders and read-back requirement, 16–17
MEDMARX database, 25
Methicillin-resistant *Staphylococcus aureus* (MRSA) infection, 12, 26
Mission and strategic planning, responsibility for, 36
Mnemonic for behavior-based safety expectations, 80
Monaco, 1
Mortality rates
decrease in and board involvement in quality and safety issues, vi, 72
infant mortality rate, 1
outcomes-of-care measure on, 7
staffing levels and, 23
Mouth, 80
MRSA (methicillin-resistant *Staphylococcus aureus*) infection, 12, 26
Multidisciplinary teams, 9
Multidrug-resistant organisms, 26, 57

N

National Association for Healthcare Quality, 11
National Committee for Quality Health Care, 6
National health care reform legislation, v, 2–4
National Hospital Inpatient Quality Measures, 50
National Patient Safety Foundation, 11
National Patient Safety Goals
applicability of, 56
basis for, 56
compliance with, information about, 4
development and implementation of, 4, 56
list of, 57–58
monitoring performance through, 86
patient education on, 60
topics for, 22, 23

National Quality Forum (NQF)
creation of, 5–6
purpose and goals of, 5–6
quality measures
development of, 6
endorsement of, 50
monitoring performance through, 86
review and possible endorsement of, 52
safe practices, 6
serious reportable events, 13
serious reportable events list, 6
Never events, 6–7, 8
New Zealand, 1
Non-accountability measures, 51–52
NQF. *See* National Quality Forum (NQF)
Nurse shortage. *See* Staffing issues
Nursing-sensitive care measures, 50, 52

O

Office of Quality Monitoring, 53–54
100,000 Lives Campaign (IHI), 11, 12
ORYX initiative
accountability measures in, 52
beginning of, 49
core measures and core measure sets, 4, 49–50
data collection through, 10
data to support Priority Focus Process, 45
general requirements of, 50–51
mandatory participation in, 51
monitoring performance through, 86
ORYX Performance Measurement Report, 51
Outcomes of care
accountability measures, 51–52
close calls and, 16
communication of, standard on, 35
data about, access to, 7
improvement of, 2, 72–73
staffing levels and, 23
Outcomes-of-care measures, 7

111

Outpatient department, hospital, core measure set on, 50
Over-the-counter medications, 25

P

Patient-centered activities, 77–78, 80, 83–84
Patients
  charity care, qualifications for, 3
  chronic conditions, care for patients with, 9
  comorbidities and medication management, 24–25
  education of, 59–60
  family members and patients
    committees, participation on, 84, 96–97
    communication with, 19–20, 43
    insight about quality and safety issues through, 91, 96–97
  identification of, 57
  insight about through patient stories, 91
  involvement in care by, 14–15, 59–60, 97
Patient safety
  involvement in by board, 11, 12, 13
  Joint Commission programs and services related to, 4
  NQF safe practices to reduce risk of harm to patients, 6
  program for, standard on, 18, 35
  staffing shortages and, 23–24
Patient Safety Leadership WalkRounds, 77
"Patient's Health Journal," 60
Pay-for-performance programs, vi
Payments
  bundled payments, 3
  CMS incentive payments program, 51
  CMS payments, decrease in, 2, 4
  CMS payment system, health care reform and, 3
  CMS reimbursements, 6
  reduced payments for higher-than-expected readmission rates, 3
  reimbursements, decrease in, v

Performance data
  collection of, 21–22
  decisions about provider preferences and, vi, 12–13
  dissemination of, 4
  Hospital Compare, 3, 7
  hospital reporting of, incentives for, 7
  physician comparison database, 3
  Premier Hospital Quality Incentive Demonstration, 79
  reimbursements and, vi
  reliability of, 21–22
  standardization of, 13
Performance improvement
  activities to support, 44
  CEO evaluation and, vi, 73, 93–95
  dashboards, vi, 72, 87
  involvement in by board, vi, 11, 12, 13, 71–72, 85–88, 97–98
  library of measures, 52
  methodology for, 21
  monitoring of, 86–87
  opportunities for, 4
  reports on initiatives, 87
  resources for, 76, 87–88, 89–90, 92–93
  Strategic Surveillance System (S3), 4, 52–53
Performance measurement. *See also* ORYX initiative
  accountability measures, 4, 51–52
  goal of, 53
  incorporation of into day-to-day activities, 10
  information about, dissemination of, 4
  involvement in by board, 85–88, 90
  Joint Commission programs and services related to, 4, 33
  library of measures, 52
  measures, recommendation of, 91–92
  National Hospital Inpatient Quality Measures, 50
  non-accountability measures, 51–52
  process for, 21–22
  reliability of, 21–22

Index

Targeted Solutions Tool for, 5
Performance Plus program, 95
Perinatal care
    core measure set, 50
    perinatal death/loss of function, 16, 55
Physicians and health care professionals
    communication between, 20–21
    communication competency requirements, 20
    compensation for, basis for, 94–95
    competence of, 9, 44
    decisions about provider preferences, performance data for, vi, 12–13
    influenza vaccinations for, 27
    physician comparison database, 3
    staffing shortages, 23–24
    training of
        in communication methods, 20
        on quality and safety principles and measures, 74
        for technology use, 26
Pneumonia
    antibiotic administration to patients with, 52
    core measure set on, 49
    influenza vaccinations for, 51
    non-accountability measures, 52
    outcomes-of-care measure on, 7
    process-of-care measure on, 7
    ventilator-associated
        causes of, 27
        prevention of, 12
Premier, Inc., 79
Premier Hospital Quality Incentive Demonstration, 79
President's Advisory Commission on Consumer Protection and Quality in the Health Care Industry, 5
Pressure ulcers
    as non-reimbursable hospital-acquired condition, 8
    prevention of, 12
    St. Vincent's Medical Center "Healthcare That Is Safer" initiative, 86
Prices for items and services, availability of, 3
Priority Focus Area Dashboard Report, 53
Priority focus areas, 45–46, 53
Priority Focus Process, 45–47, 52, 53
Priority Focus Process Reports, 46
Processes and systems
    changes in to support performance improvement, 44
    design of, standard on, 35, 44
    errors and system failures, 16–17
    improvement of, 21
    proactive approach to prevention of errors related to system failures, 17–21
    safety and quality focus of, standard related to, 21
    staff role in evaluation on, 24
    technology use and, 26
Process-of-care measures, 7
Program-specific tracers, 48
Project Zero, 88, 89–90, 91
Provena Saint Joseph Medical Center
    emergency department initiative, 85
    performance improvement initiatives, 92
Psychiatric services, hospital-based inpatient, core measure set on, 50
Public Company Accounting Reform and Investor Protection Act (Sarbanes-Oxley Act), 14
Public policy initiatives, 4
Pulmonary embolism, 8

Q

Quality and safety
    accountability for, 77, 84–85, 91–92, 93–95
    barriers to, Targeted Solutions Tool to identify, 5
    behavior-based safety expectations, 80
    board meetings, discussions about during, 72, 95–97
    CMS's role in, 6
    common areas of concern, 22–28

communication and, 19–21
communication between leaders about, 40–41
complaints or concerns about, process for reporting, 53–54
culture of safety and quality
  communication and, 20
  creation of, 17–18
  promotion of, 73–75, 78, 80
  standard related to, 18, 41–42
familiarity with issues, 1, 15, 71
Hospital Quality and Safety Survey (Leapfrog Group), 10–11
improvement of
  board's role in, 71–74
  focus on, 44
information related to, communication of (LD.03.04.01), 43
Institute of Medicine reports on, 7, 9–10
involvement in by board, vi, 11, 12, 13, 71–72, 97–98
Joint Commission programs and services related to, 4
national commitment to improvement of, 5–6
national health care reform legislation and, v
performance reports on, vi
planning activities to support, 43
priority of, vi
processes and systems that focus on, standard related to, 21
quality measures, development of, 3
ranking of U.S. on metrics related to, 1
resources for, 76, 87–88, 89–90
responsibility for, v–vi, 36, 38–39, 71–72, 97–98
staffing for, 44
training on quality and safety principles and measures, vi, 74
Quality Check
  accountability measures information on, 52
  information available through, 60

information dissemination through, 4
patient education on, 60
Quality committees and subcommittees, vi, 72, 73, 95–96
Quality dashboards, vi, 72, 87
Quality Monitoring, Office of, 53–54
Quality Monitoring System database, 45
Quality Report, 60–69

R

Radiation, exposure to, 7, 55
Rape, 16, 55
Readmission rates
  interventions to decrease, 2
  outcomes-of-care measure on, 7
  reduced payments for higher-than-expected rates, 3
Recession, v
Resources for improvement activities, 76, 87–88, 89–90, 92–93
Restraints, death and injury in, 16
Rewarding Results initiative, 11
Robert Wood Johnson Foundation, 11
Robust Process Improvement (RPI) methods, 5, 22, 58
Root causes analysis, 17, 90
RPI (Robust Process Improvement) methods, 5, 22, 58

S

Safety. *See* Patient safety; Quality and safety
St. Luke's Hospital performance monitoring dashboards and reports, 87
St. Vincent's Medical Center "Healthcare That Is Safer" initiative, 86
Sarbanes-Oxley Act (Public Company Accounting Reform and Investor Protection Act), 14
Securities and Exchange Commission, 14
Sentara Healthcare
  compensation for employees, basis for, 94, 95

Index

Performance Plus program, 95
quality subcommittee policy, 72
walkarounds program, 80
Sentinel Event Alert, 4, 55–56
Sentinel Event Database, 4, 17, 54–55, 56
Sentinel events
   definition of, 15, 55
   errors compared to, 16
   informing board of investigations and their outcome, 15
   reporting errors related to, 16
   reporting of, 16–17, 54
   reviewable events, 17, 54, 55
   root causes analysis, 17, 90
   Sentinel Event Policy, 17, 54–56
   top 10 types reported, 16
Serious reportable events, 6, 13
Singapore, 1
Six Sigma, 5, 22
Smart Parent's Guide to Getting Your Kids Through Checkups, Illnesses, and Accidents (Joint Commission and JCR), 60
Smart pumps, 25
Smoking cessation counseling, 52
Speak Up (Joint Commission), 15, 59
Speak Up program, 59
Staff. *See* Physicians and health care professionals
Staffing issues
   effective staffing, 23
   health care staffing services certification, 34
   job satisfaction and productivity and, 24
   patient safety risks and, 23–24
   prevalence of staffing shortages, 23–24
   quality and safety, staffing for, 44
   recruitment and retention of staff, 24
   staffing shortages, 23–24
   strategies to address shortages, 24
Standards
   compliance with, information about, 4
   development of, 33, 35
   focus of, 35–36
   revision of, 36
Strategic Surveillance System (S3), 4, 52–53
Strokes
   core measure set on, 50
   process-of-care measure on, 7
Suicides, 16, 55, 56, 57, 92
Surgical Care Improvement Project, 12, 50
Surgical procedures
   antibiotic administration prior to, 51–52
   complications, operative and postoperative, 16
   foreign object retained after, 8, 16, 55
   infections after surgery, process-of-care measure on, 7
   surgical site infections
      causes of, 27
      as nonreimbursable hospital-acquired condition, 8
      prevention of, 12, 57
      quality solution for, 5
      targeted solutions for, 58
   Universal Protocol for Preventing Wrong Site, Wrong Procedure, Wrong Person Surgery, 56, 57, 60
   wrong-site surgery
      quality solutions for, 5
      as reviewable event, 55
      as sentinel event, 16
      targeted solutions for, 58
Surveys
   initial surveys, 48
   involvement in by board, 83
   leadership session, 83
   Priority Focus Process and, 45–47, 52, 53
   tracer methodology, 48–49
   unannounced surveys, 47–48
System tracers, 49

T

Targeted solutions
   definition of, 23
   development of, 23, 33
   for hand hygiene compliance, 27

for hand-off communication, 23
Targeted Solutions Tool, 5, 23, 27, 58
Teams and teamwork
    collaborative relationships, 18, 20, 24
    multidisciplinary teams, 9
    standard related to, 42
Technology
    automation of clinical information, 9, 25–26
    implementation challenges, 26
    for medication management, 25–26
    training in use of, 26
Test results
    computerized notification of critical, 25
    timely reporting of, 57
Tobacco core measure set, 50
To Err Is Human (Institute of Medicine), 7, 9, 10, 14–15
Tracer methodology, 48–49
Transfusion errors and reactions, 8, 55, 57
Trauma and falls, 8
20 Tips to Help Prevent Medical Errors (Agency for Healthcare Research and Quality), 15

U

Unannounced surveys, 47–48
United Kingdom, 1
United States Department of Defense facilities, 48
United States Department of Health and Human Services, 2, 3, 35
Universal precautions, 27
Universal Protocol for Preventing Wrong Site, Wrong Procedure, Wrong Person Surgery, 56, 57, 60
Urinary tract infections, catheter-associated, 8, 27

V

Vaccinations, influenza, 27, 51
Value-based services, payment for, 3
Vancomycin-resistant enterococci, 26
Vascular catheter–associated infection. *See* Central line infections
Venous thromboembolism, core measure set on, 50
Verbal orders and read-back requirement, 16–17
Veterans Health Administration, 11
Violence in health care settings, 56

W

Walkarounds, 77–78, 80, 83–84
World Health Organization (WHO) hand-hygiene guidelines, compliance with, 57
Wrong-site surgery
    quality solutions for, 5
    as reviewable event, 55
    as sentinel event, 16
    targeted solutions for, 58
    Universal Protocol for Preventing Wrong Site, Wrong Procedure, Wrong Person Surgery, 56, 57, 60

Y

YOU: The Smart Patient (Joint Commission), 15, 59–60